DO IT YOURSELF

A Complete Guide to Wet Cupping

Included Are Cupping Points Illustrations For 94 Types of Diseases

DISCLAIMER

You do not have the right to resell or give this book/e-book for free to others.

This book/e-book is the copyright of the writer, any form of reproduction without permission either electronically or physically is prohibited.

Legal Notice: The e-book and cupping guide video are made based on the writer's experience in the field of cupping treatment. The writer has gone through the course in cupping and is using the right techniques. The writer is not responsible for any mistakes or accidents that occur during the process of cupping. If you have any problem and are unsure of the explanations in the e-book and cupping guide video, please email to aswadi.aziz@yahoo.com

Contents

1. The history of cupping

2. What is cupping?

3. Types of cupping

4. Benefits and advantages of cupping

5. Diseases that can be healed with cupping

6. The best time for cupping?

7. Prohibitions in cupping

8. Propositions on the need for cupping

9. Methods of cupping

      i.   Tools used

      ii.   How the cupping treatment is done

      iii.   Recommended cupping points according to diseases

THE HISTORY OF CUPPING

Cupping has been known since the time of Prophet Musa a.s. It is a process of sucking or removing blood from the body with a cup through the surface of the skin. It is also more practical, without side effects, cheap and able to treat diseases that cannot be cured with modern medication.

Cupping is a very effective method of eliminating pain and restoring the immune system. It is actually a technique that can induce the inactive or weak nerves, and through this way the body system will stimulate and improve the immune system.

Keys to Being Healthy
1. Taking care of health and eating healthy food.
2. Striving to prevent the spread of diseases and everything that is harmful to health.
3. Removing damaging elements in the body such as toxic, vomit, vapours and dirty blood.

Causes of Diseases

Diseases are caused by the blood that is no longer functional in the body. Eventually it becomes poisonous and reduces the body's fitness. If it is not eliminated, the body cannot survive due to the toxin (impurity or poisoning). Thus, diseases such as kidney problems, diabetes, hypertension and other harmful diseases will transpire.

What is cupping?

Cupping is a medical treatment of the Prophet Muhammad (peace be upon him; pbuh) that has been modernised following the scientific methods to remove harmful toxic wastes from the body through the skin surface.

This is one of the ways of effective 'Detoxification' (toxic removal) that is safe with no side effects. A lot of toxic is accumulated underneath the skin as it is the biggest organ in the body.

Cupping is very effective in relieving or eliminating pain, restoring body function, as well as giving hopes to patients to continuously seek treatment.

Cupping in the Malay term is 'Bekam' which means "Release of Blood", and is known as "Cupping" in English. In Arabic, it is translated as "al-Hijamah".

A healthy body and an intelligent mind are important factors in a person's life in order to carry out his life responsibilities. However, if there is too much toxic in his body, it can cause 'Blood Stasis' or 'Hematostatic Blood', in which the blood system does not flow smoothly.

This condition will disrupt the physical and mental health little by little. The characteristics that will appear if a person has too much toxic in his body are laziness, depression, always complaining of being unwell, easily bored and irritable.

The Nature of Blood with Cupping

1. Blood undergoes oxidation without air.
2. The plasma separates itself from the blood.
3. The blood that is accumulated is one-tenth of the rate of the white blood cells that is present in the natural blood (Enhances body immunity).
4. At the peak of red blood cells, all white blood cells have an odd shape. This means that the content is unable to carry out its functions to the extent it can eliminate dirty red blood cells and unwanted blood with the remainder being white blood.

Differences between Cupping and Blood Donation

Cupping
- Blood is from capillaries
- Removing toxins and dirt only
- No Withdrawal of White Blood Cells
- Only LDL Withdrawal – Withdrawal of HDL and LDL
- Excessive emission of iron on the skin

Blood Donation

- Blood is from veins.
- Outflow of all fluid content
- Issuing of white blood cells red blood cells
- Issuing of HDL and LDL
- Removing minerals and iron in the body

Importance of Cupping

The body has 3 mechanisms of eliminating toxins in it which are the excretion of faeces and urine and sweat through skin (Recreation), so if one of the discharge mechanism is problematic, it will cause a toxin build-up disturbance in a particular area. Skin is the largest area to remove toxins through natural sweating in which the toxins in the body will be pushed up to the surface of the skin.

If the toxins on the top of the skin are not removed properly, the accumulation of toxins on the area will occur causing the flow of energy, blood, lymph nodes and nerves, also causing it to interfere with the places that the path (Meridian) will pass.

Types of Cupping

Currently, there are many types of cupping available due to the existence of various equipment and ideas.

1) **Wet Cupping**

   This is the type of cupping that will be practised in the e-book and cupping guide video. This is the Sunnah cupping as practised by Rasulullah. Whoever that practises this type of cupping will be rewarded accordingly for practising the Sunnah of Rasulullah. This type of cupping involves the use of equipment and the process of removing blood will take place.

2) **Dry Cupping**

   Wind cupping is a process to remove wind from the body by means of using the equipment for blood cupping, but it does not involve the use of cupping knife or needle. This type of cupping does not involve the issuing of blood.

3) **Leech Cupping**

   Leech cupping is similar to blood cupping as it involves the removal of blood. However, it does not involve the use of cupping equipment. It uses leeches as the toxin blood sucker.

Benefits and Advantages of Cupping

1) Removing stress, exhaustion and shoulder and neck pain
2) Earning rewards for practising the Sunnah of the Prophet Muhammad
3) Treating witchcraft problems. (will be discussed in the chapter on treating witchcraft)

Diseases that can be healed with cupping

Preventing and healing various diseases with Allah's will such as:

- Obesity
- Elephantiasis
- Sciatica
- Stomach ache
- Constipation
- Heart & Gastric Disorders
- Reduced Rib Function, Inflammation and Pain Function
- Food Allergy
- Bone Sore
- Breathing Difficulty
- Asthma
- Insomnia

- Diarrhoea
- Muscle Cramp
- Diabetes
- Gall Bladder and Liver Disorders
- Shivering Without Fever
- Bed-wetting
- Tonsil
- Itchiness
- Colon Inflammation
- Stress
- Bladder Disorder
- Irregular Period
- Kidney
- Hypertension
- Knee Pain
- Pain in the Legs
- Pain Around the Spine
- Mental Disorder
- Paralysed due to Blockage of Brain Blood Vessels (Stroke)
- Gout
- Rheumatoid
- Wounds, Boils on the Calf and Buttocks
- Decreased Body Endurance
- Sinus
- Pain in the Stomach Area
- Rib Disorder and Rib Skin Disease
- Haemorrhoids
- Heart Disease
- Infertility
- Excessive Sleeping
- Migraine
- Improve Blood Circulation
- Narrow and Clogged Blood Vessels

- Sore Buttocks
- Shoulder and Neck Pain
- Shoulder Pain
- Skinny Body
- Help Quit Smoking
- Hearing Problem, Inflammation and Ear Swelling
- Infection of Germs
- Improve Blood Circulation
- Decreased Blood Flow
- Improve Memory
- Improve Concentration
- Anal Fistula
- Waist Pain
- Bladder Disorder
- Pins and Needles in the Legs
- Pins and Needles in the Hands
- Muscle Pull (Sprain)
- Full Paralysis
- Dizziness due to Stomach Disorder or Constipation
- Prostate Disorder and Impotence
- Dizziness due to Backbone Disorder
- Bladder and Liver Disorders
- Dizziness during Menstruation for Women
- Pain in the Thigh and Soles of the Feet
- Cold on the Soles of the Feet
- Nervous (Tense / Restless)
- Brain Tumour
- Thickening and Hardening of the Soles of the Feet
- Numb Knees
- Pancreas Disorder
- Cramps
- Unable to Speak
- Eye Disease

- Weak Brain Cells Function
- Ceased Menstruation
- Testis Swelling
- Low Blood Pressure
- Various Womb Diseases
- Discharge of Vaginal Fluid Without Smell, Colour and Itchiness
- Discharge of Vaginal Fluid
- Trigeminus and Facial Nerve Inflammation
- Improve Egg Productivity (Fertility)
- Dizziness due to Tired Eyes
- Chronic Coughing and Lung Diseases
- Headache and Drowsiness due to High Blood Pressure
- Headache due to Inflammation Around the Nasal Cavity
- Dizziness due to Anaemia
- Dizziness due to Influenza

The Best Time for Cupping

There is no specific date and time for cupping, but it is recommended to be most suitably done on the 17th, 19th and 21st of the month according to the Islamic calendar. It is also recommended to have an empty stomach before cupping.

Prohibitions in Cupping

1. Diabetics are not encouraged to do wet cupping unless it is done by an expert and experienced person in cupping.
2. Do not do cupping on people who are physically weak and tired (over fatigue).
3. Do not do cupping on people who suffer from uneven skin diseases or severe skin allergies such as ulceration and oedema.
4. Do not do cupping on physically weak people and weak children or children under 3 years of age.
5. Leukaemia patients (blood cancer) are not encouraged to do wet cupping.

6. Patients with severe hepatitis, active TBC, haemophilia, malignant anaemia, thrombocytopenia and other critical diseases are not encouraged to do cupping unless it is done by an expert and experienced person in cupping.

7. Do not do cupping on: Full stomach, thirstiness, hunger, fatigue, after heavy work, weak body and feverish body (coldness).

8. Do not do cupping on pregnant women who are in the first 3 months (early trimester).

9. Do not do cupping on wounds, torn joints, fractures, varicose veins, tumours.

10. Do not do cupping on menstruating and puerperal women.

11. Do not do cupping on the hardened part of the stomach.

12. Do not do cupping immediately after eating, it can be done two hours after eating. Do not immediately eat after cupping, take only sweet drinks like honey or others.

13. People with heart disease are not encouraged to do cupping, unless it is under the supervision of a doctor or an expert and experienced person in cupping.

14. Do not do cupping immediately after bath, especially after bathing with cold water. It is not encouraged to immediately bathe after cupping, but it can be done after 2 hours. It is encouraged to bathe with hot/warm water.

15. People who have just donated blood or involved in an accident are not advised to do wet cupping as it can cause reduction of blood.

16. Do not do cupping on diabetics (blood sugar above 280) unless by an expert.

17. Do not do cupping in an open space or a cold place. It is best to do it at a warm place or a place with the normal temperature.

Prohibited Body Parts for Cupping

1. Natural holes of the body:

   - Eyes
   - Nose
   - Ears
   - Mouth
   - Genitals
   - Anus
   - Nipples

2. The area of lymph nodes system that functions as a producer of antibodies, that is in the submaxillary, korvikal, sudmalaonkular, axillary, heart rate section, inguinalglimfa nodes.

3. Areas that are close to the large vessels.

Propositions on the need for Cupping

1) Prophet Muhammad pbuh said, "If there is a medicine to heal diseases, then cupping can also cure them." — Reported by Malik

2) Prophet Muhammad pbuh said, "I did not pass by any group on the night when I was taken on the Night Journey (Isra'), but they said to me, 'O Muhammad, tell your ummah to do cupping." — Reported by Ibnu Majah

3) Prophet Muhammad pbuh said, "Healing is to be found in three things: drinking honey, the knife of the cupper, and cauterization of fire, but I forbid my followers to use cauterization (branding with fire)." — Reported by Al Bukhari

Frequently Asked Questions

1) Is the method of blood cupping painful?
No, because the method of blood cupping nowadays uses a type of tool called the CUPPING PEN. The pinprick made on the skin by this pen is extremely fast that it makes you unaware that the pinprick is made to your skin. The method of this pinprick is similar to the method used for blood test and diabetes test.

2) Is it safe to do the blood cupping method?
Yes, it is because it uses a disposable lancet (needle) in which whenever it is done, a new lancet/needle will be used.

3) What is the ideal date to do blood cupping that is able to provide the maximum healing?

The ideal dates for cupping are on the 17th, 19th and 21st of the month according to the Islamic calendar, and the stomach must be empty before doing the cupping.

4) Which individuals are strictly prohibited from doing blood cupping? Individuals who are strictly prohibited from doing blood cupping are those who are very weak physically, sick elderly people, people with leukaemia, people with serious low blood pressure, people with serious skin disease and pregnant women in the first 3 months.

5) Which method of cupping provides the maximum healing?
Blood cupping method is the method that provides the maximum healing to patients generally.

6) Which method of cupping gives the Sunnah rewards when doing it? Blood cupping method.

7) How often should we go for the treatment of blood cupping?
For healthy people, they are recommended to go once a month and people with health issues are recommended to do cupping once a week for three consecutive sessions.

8) What are the prohibitions after cupping?
You are advised not to eat, bathe and sleep after the cupping treatment. You can only eat/sleep after 2 hours.

9) What is the tip before doing blood cupping?
It is recommended to fast one day before the cupping appointment or the stomach must be empty 2 hours before doing the cupping.

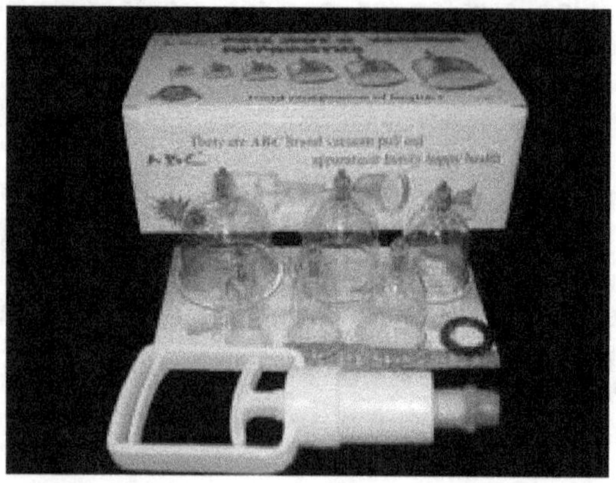

A set of cupping equipment including cups and vacuum pumps.

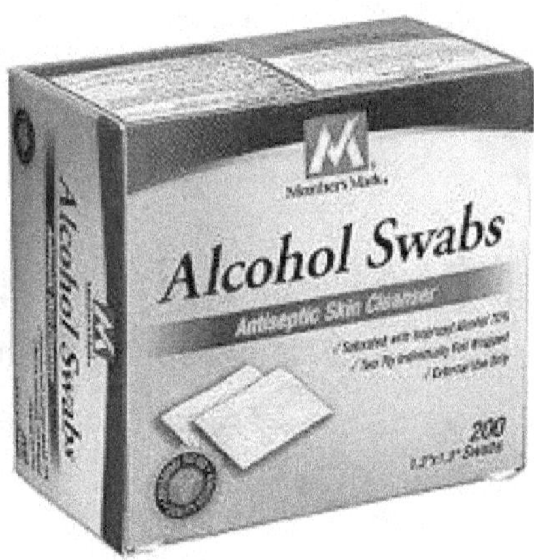

Alcohol swab (to sterilise the cupping body area)

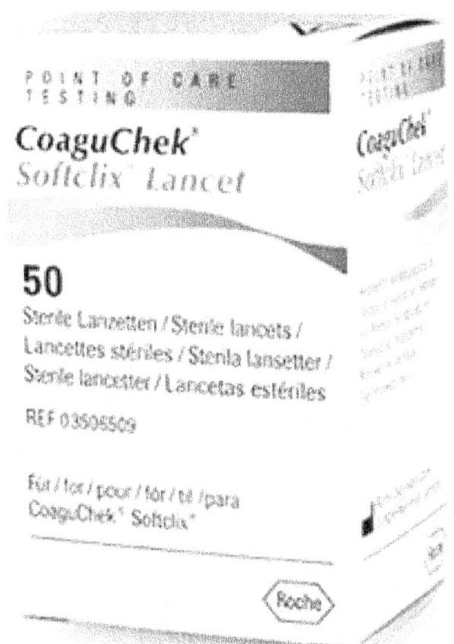

Disposable needles (lancet)

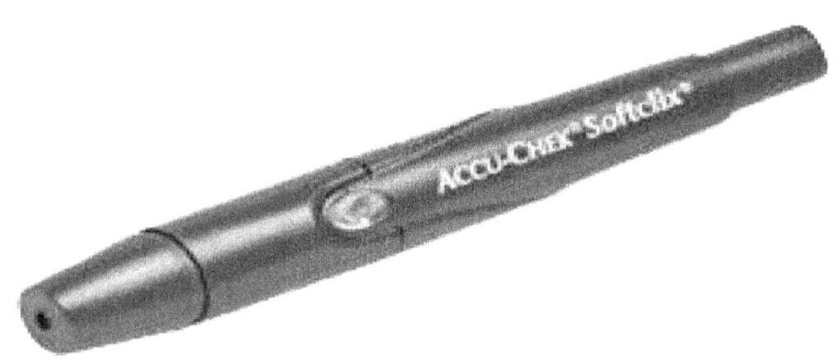

Cupping pen

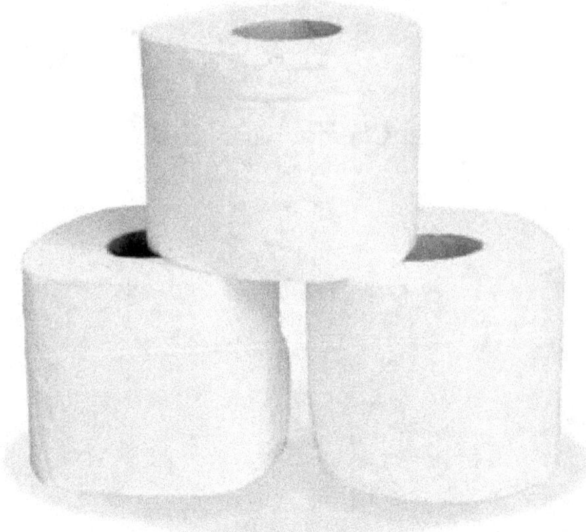

Tissue

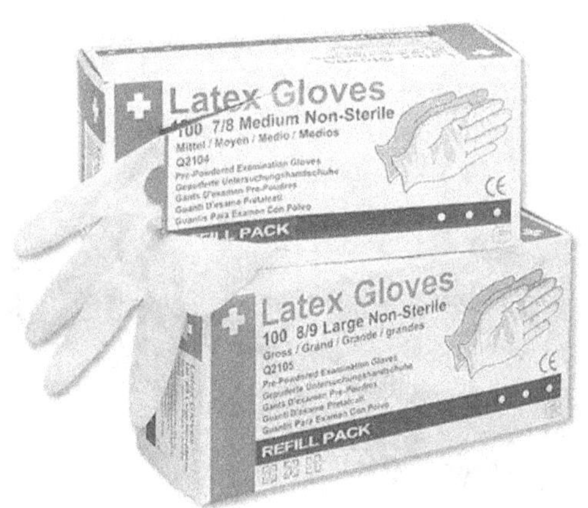

Latex gloves

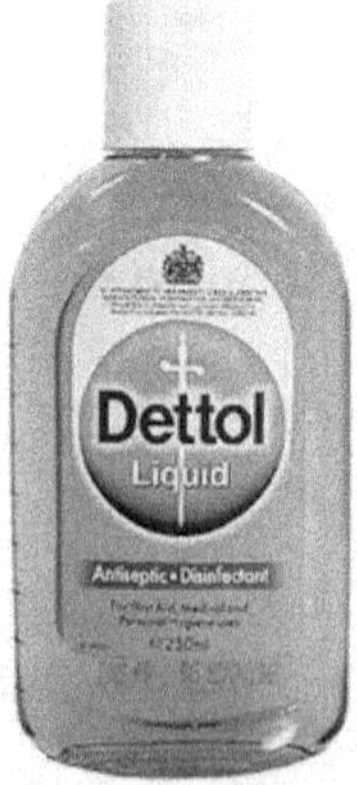

Dettol liquid (to soak/sterilise the set of cupping equipment after use)

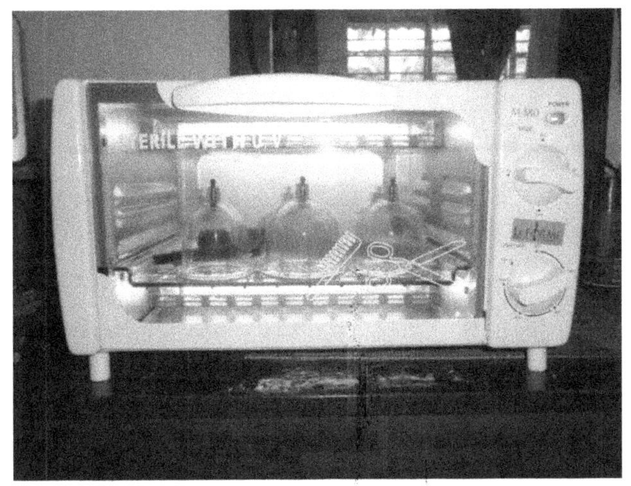

If you can afford it, you can purchase a UV Sterilizers tool to sterilise the cupping equipment.

How the Cupping Treatment is done

Step 1 (for Muslim)

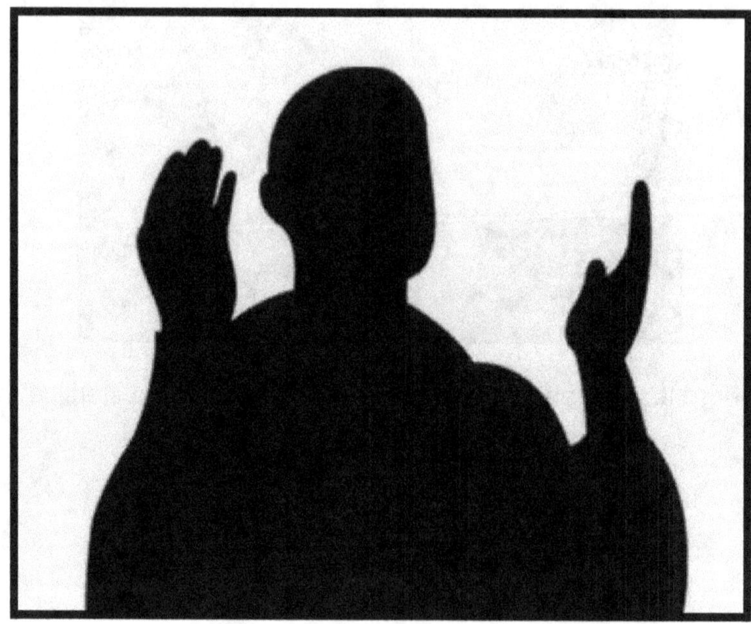

Start with reading:
1. Al-fatihah
2. 3 Qul (important if the cupping is done on a person who has been hit by witchcraft)
3. Invocation for the Prophet Muhammad
4. Syifa* invocation

اَللَّهُمَّ صَلِّ عَلَى سَيِّدِنَا مُحَمَّدٍ طِبِّ ٱلْقُلُوبِ وَدَوَآئِهَا، وَعَافِيَةِ
ٱلْأَبْدَانِ وَشِفَآئِهَا، وَنُورِ ٱلْأَبْصَارِ وَضِيَآئِهَا، وَعَلَى ءَالِهِ
وَصَحْبِهِ وَبَارِكْ وَسَلِّمْ.

Terjemahan Selawat Syifa'

Ya Allah, berilah rahmat ke atas penghulu kami, nabi Muhammad S.A.W. yang dengan berkat berselawat ke atas baginda, akan menyembuhkan hati-hati, menjadi penawar dan menyihatkan tubuh badan juga memberi kesembuhan penyakit serta mengurniakan cahaya penglihatan dan kurniakanlah juga rahmat keberkatan dan kesejahteraan ke atas keluarga dan sahabat baginda.

Translation of Syifa' Invocation:
O Allah, send blessings on our leader Muhammad, the medicine of hearts and their cure, the health of bodies and their healing, the light of eyes and their illumination, and upon his family, companions, and send peace.

Step 2

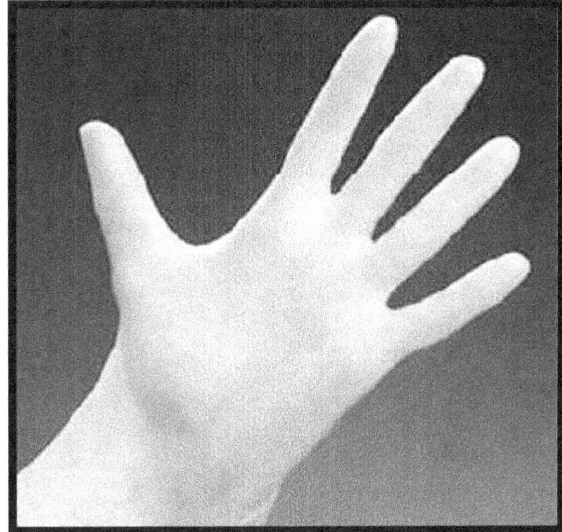

Put on the latex glove on the left hand first.

Step 3

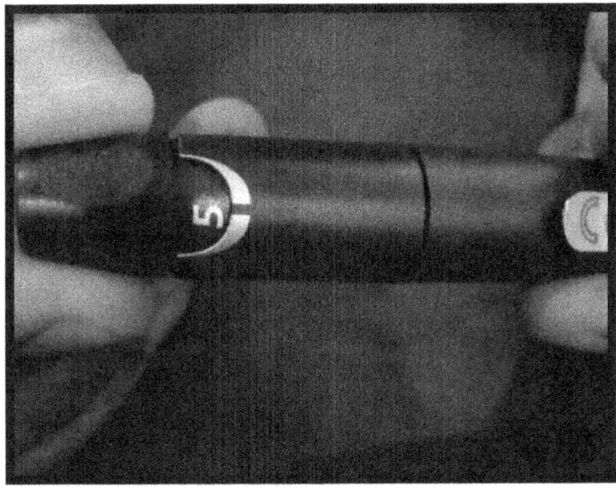

Place the lancet on the cupping pen and set the pen at level 5.

Step 4

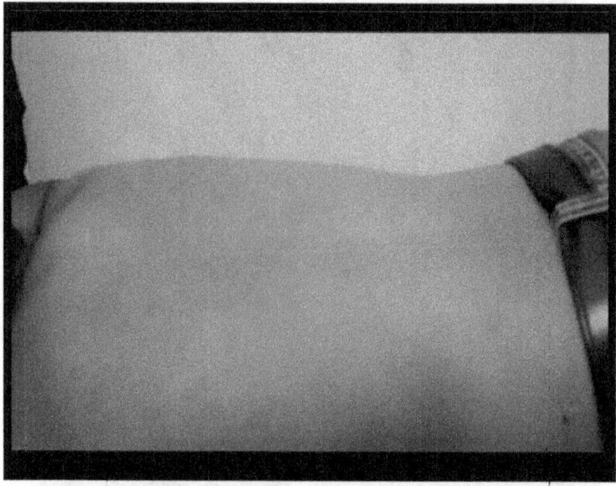

Patient lies face down or sits.

Step 5

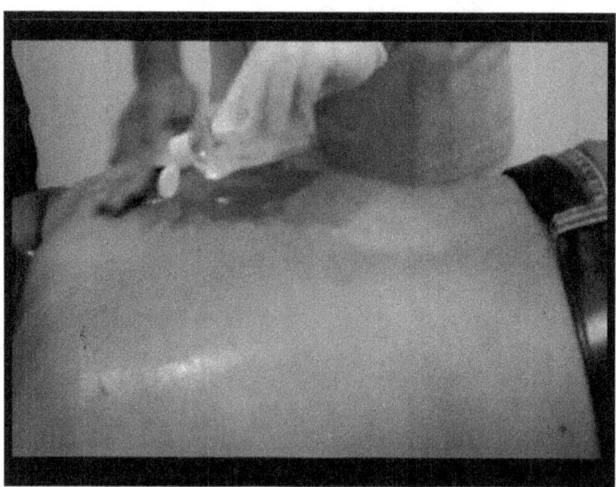

Rub and massage on the skin area that will be cupped using Baby Johnson's oil or olive oil for 10 seconds.

Step 6

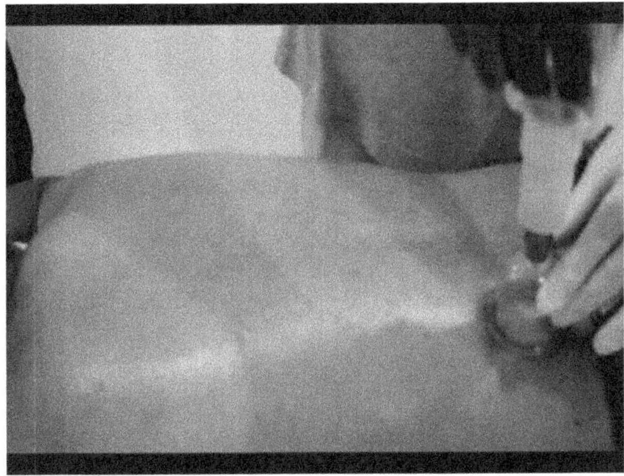

Place the cup on the surface of the skin that will be cupped. The cupping trigger is pulled 3 times.

Step 7

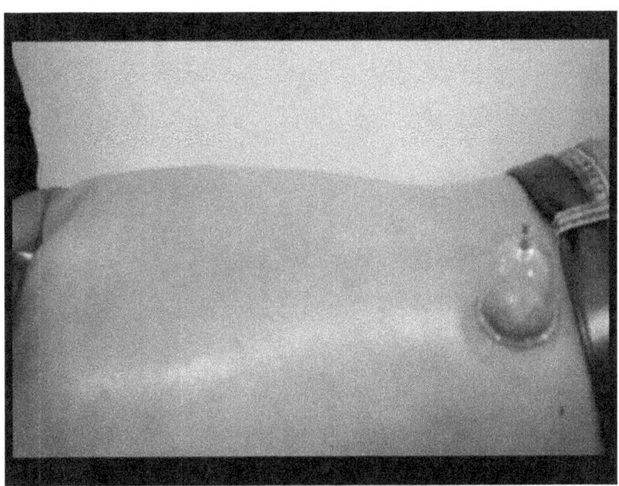

Separate the cupping cup and cupping pump and leave it for 2 minutes to give the numbness feel on the skin and to create a circled area for lancet pinpricking.

Step 8

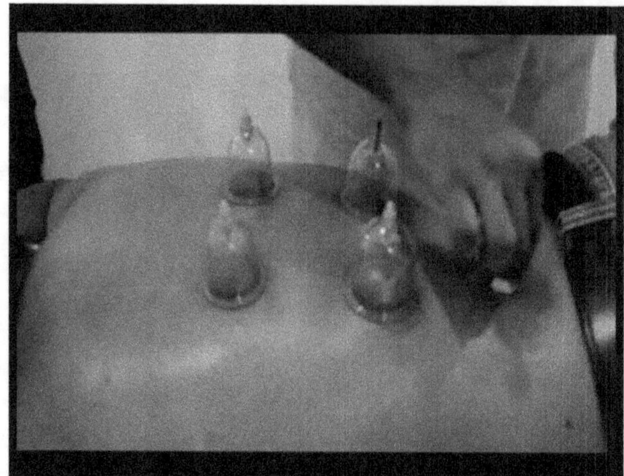

1) Pull the small button over the cupping cup to detach the cupping cup from the skin.
2) Open the alcohol swab and rub it on the skin area that will be cupped.

Step 9

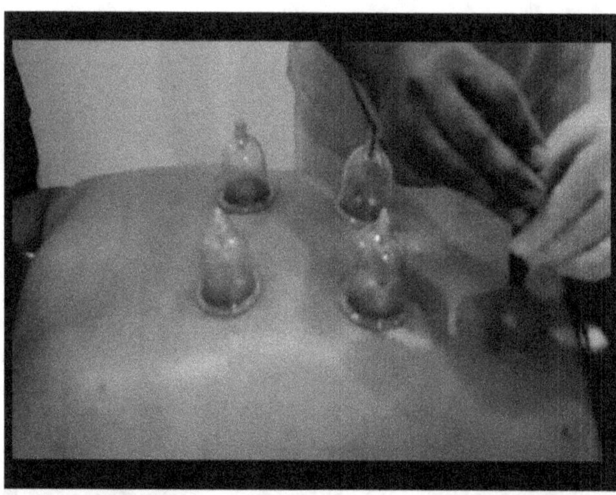

Take the cupping pen that has been placed with the lancet and pinprick evenly 30 times on the marked skin area.

Step 10

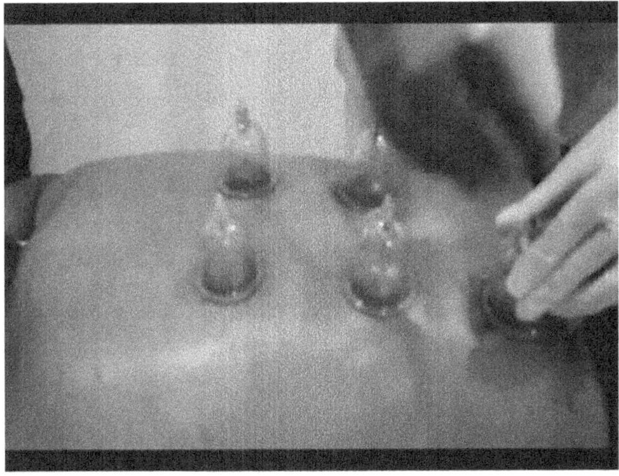

Put the cupping cup again and pull the trigger of the cupping pump 3 times also. Separate the cupping cup and the cupping pump. Leave the cupping cup for 5 minutes.

Step 11

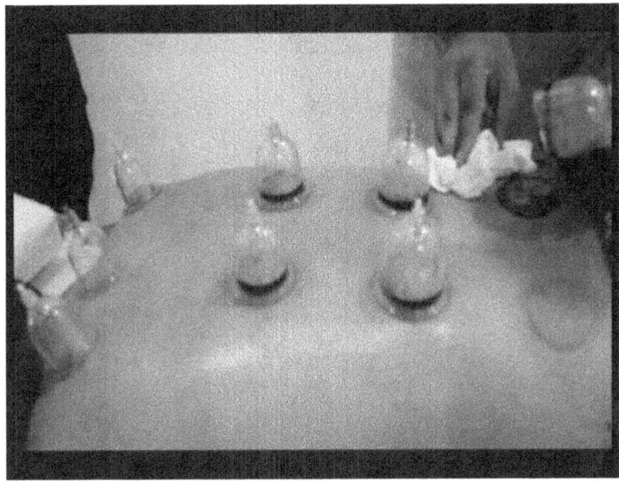

After 5 minutes, pull the cupping cup and wipe the dirty blood on the skin using tissue.

Step 12

Repeat the cupping process once more by pinpricking evenly on the same areas. Put the cupping cup again and pull the trigger of the cupping pump 3 times also for the second process of dirty blood removal.

Step 13

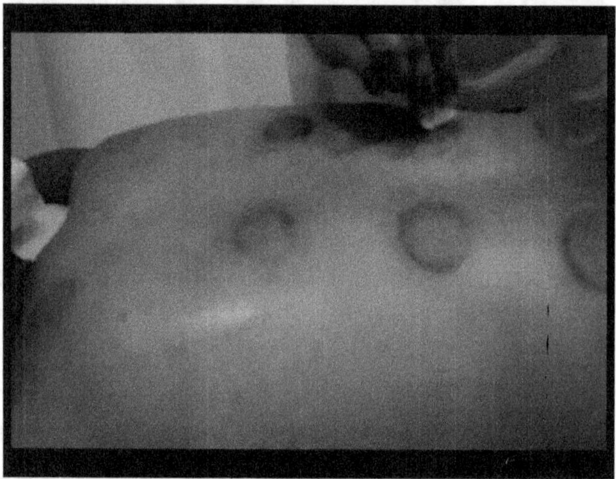

Open the alcohol swab and rub it on the skin areas that have been cupped.

Step 14

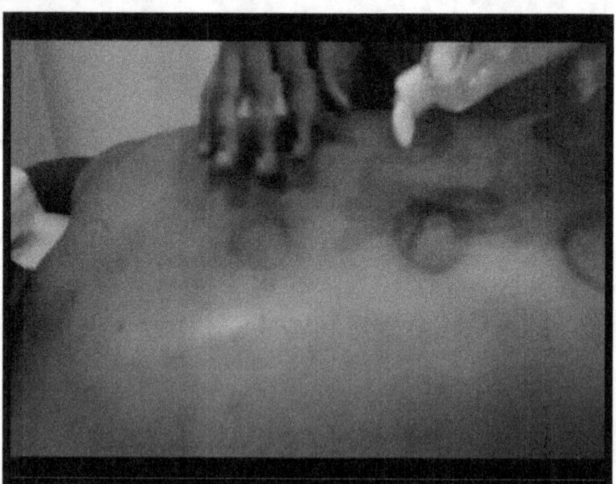

Massage all parts of the skin that have been cupped with olive oil or baby oil to reduce the effects of bruising after cupping.

Step 15

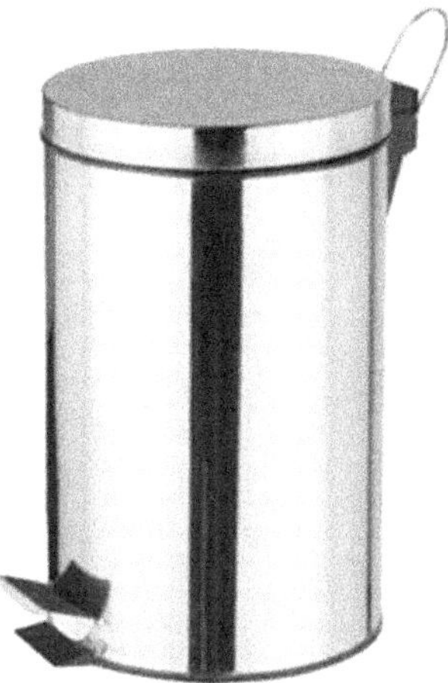

Dispose the lancet, gloves and dirty blood into the dustbin.

Step 16

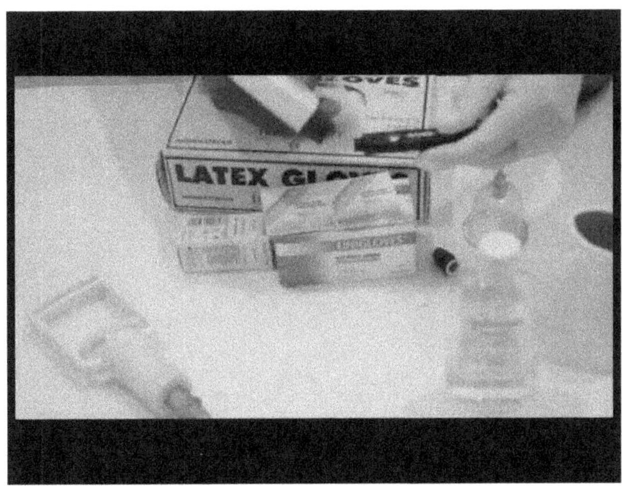

Clean the tip of the cupping pen (the area where the lancet is placed) with Dettol to disinfect.

Step 17

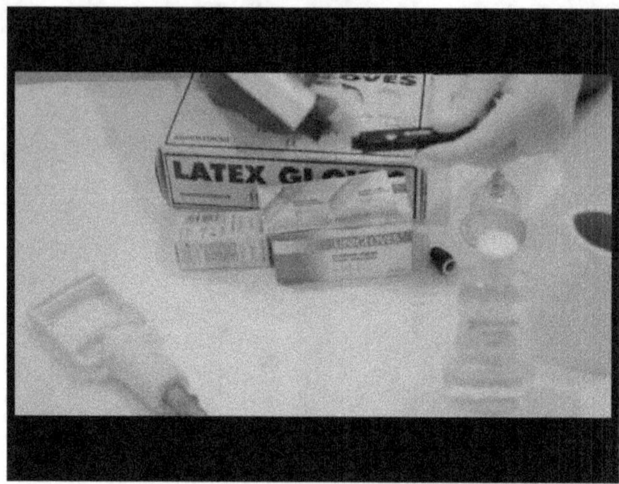

Clean the tip of the cupping pen (the area where the lancet is placed) with Dettol to disinfect.

Step 18

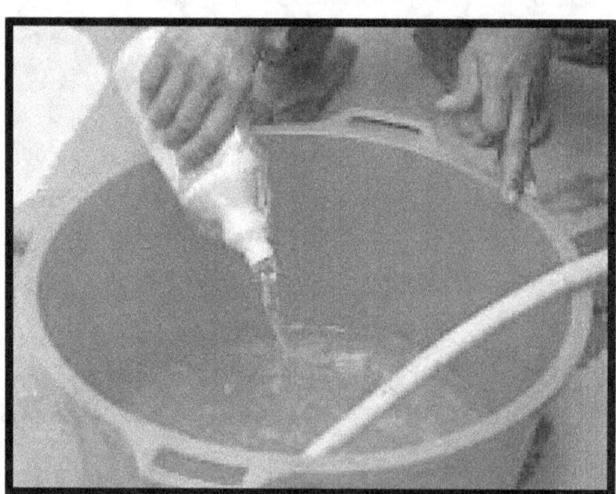

Soak and clean all the cupping equipment set involved with Dettol liquid for sterilisation purposes. Use the UV Sterilizers to sterilise if you have one.

RECOMMENDED CUPPING POINTS ACCORDING TO DISEASES

1) Cupping for Witchcraft Treatment

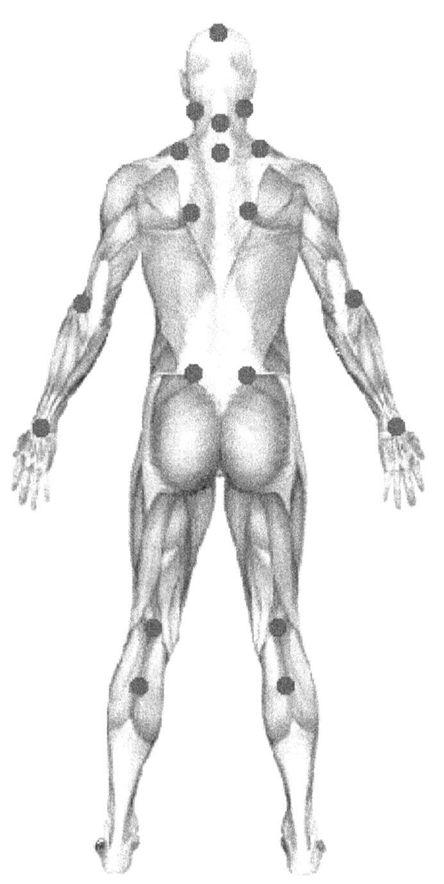

19 Cupping Points

This cupping is done after the patient has been treated with the Islamic method of treatment which is 'ruqyah'. After the completion of the 'ruqyah' method, it is recommended for the patient to do cupping once a week to remove the remainder of the poison that is left in the body by the witchcraft.

2) Cupping of the Thibbun Nabawi Sunnah

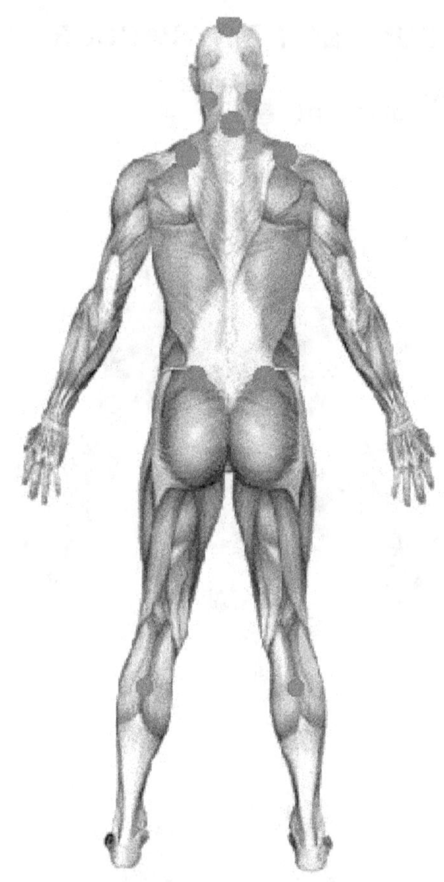

10 Cupping Points

3) Cupping for Stress/Lethargy/Fatigue Treatment

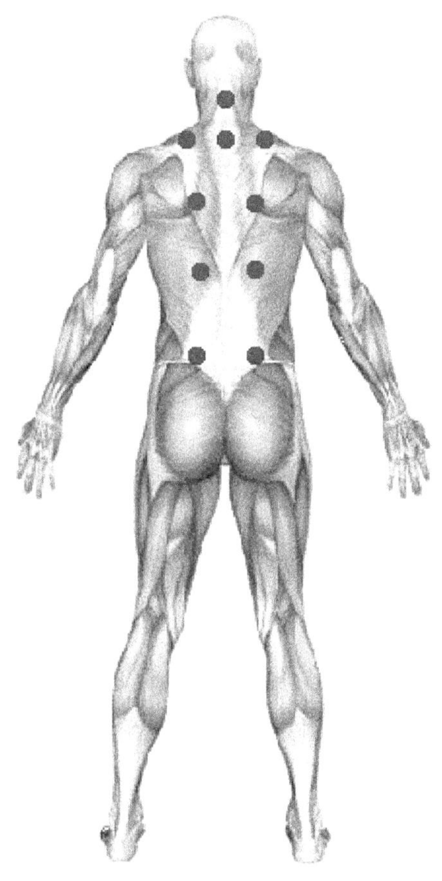

10 Cupping Points

4) Cupping for Obesity

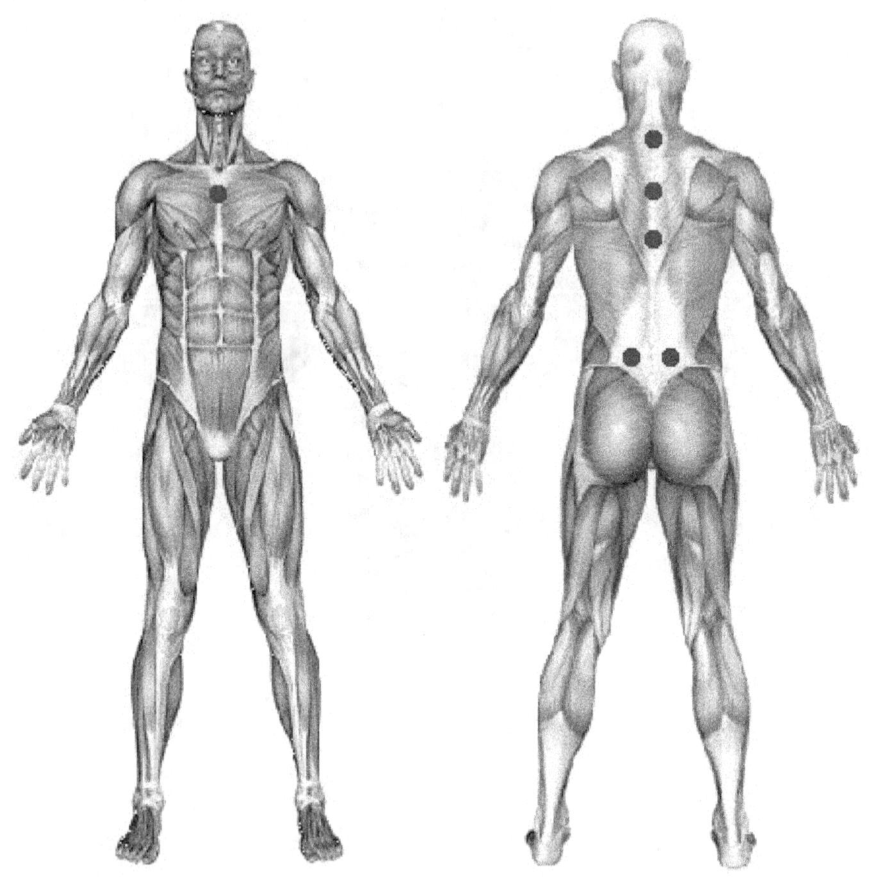

6 Cupping Points

5) Overhaul Cupping

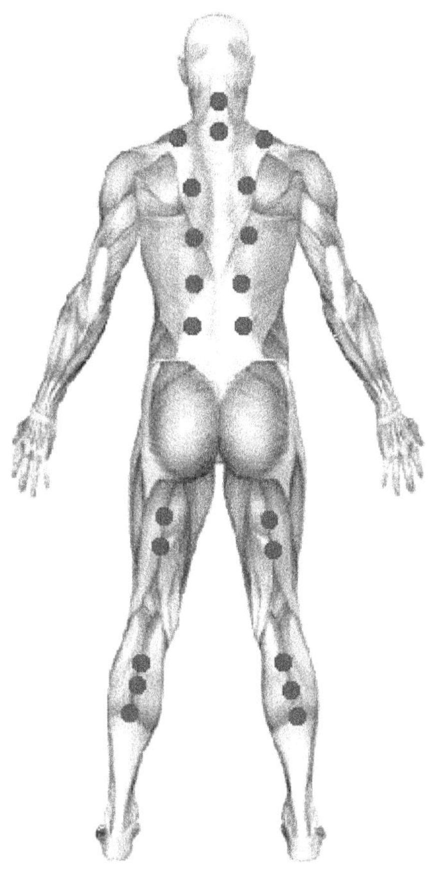

22 Cupping Points

6) Cupping for Waist Pain

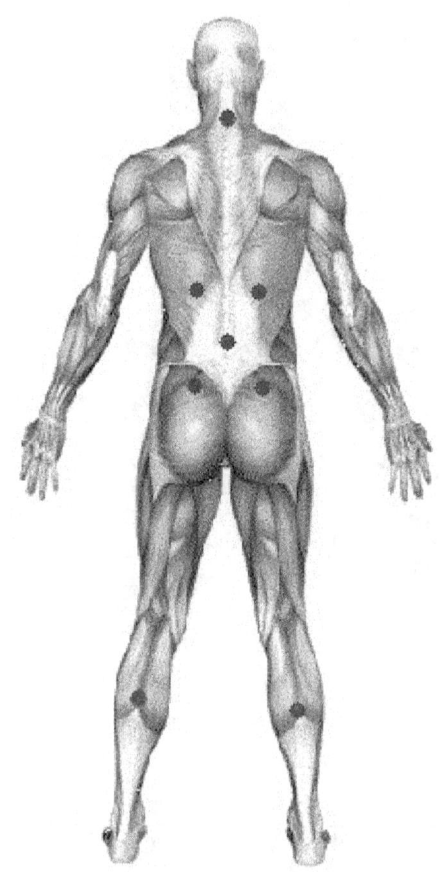

8 Cupping Points

7) Cupping for Constipation

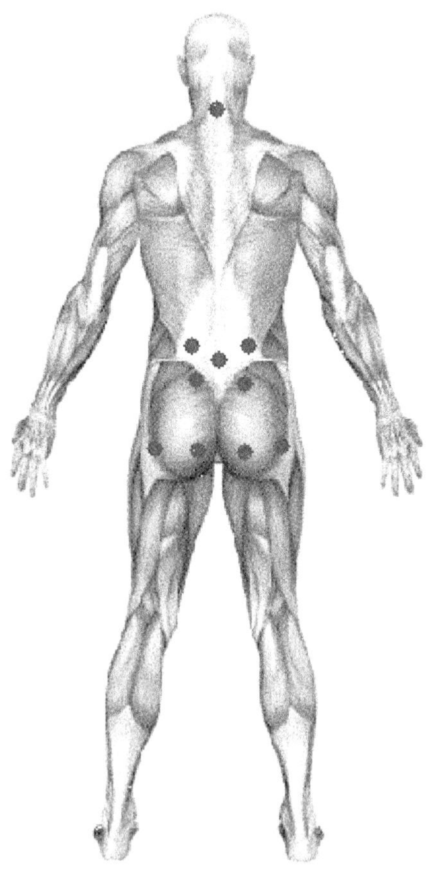

10 Cupping Points

8) Cupping for Stomach ache

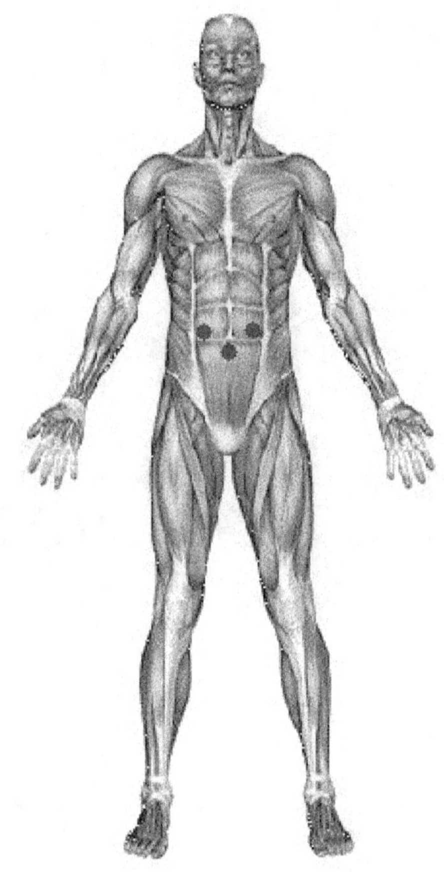

3 Cupping Points

9) Cupping for Heart Disorder

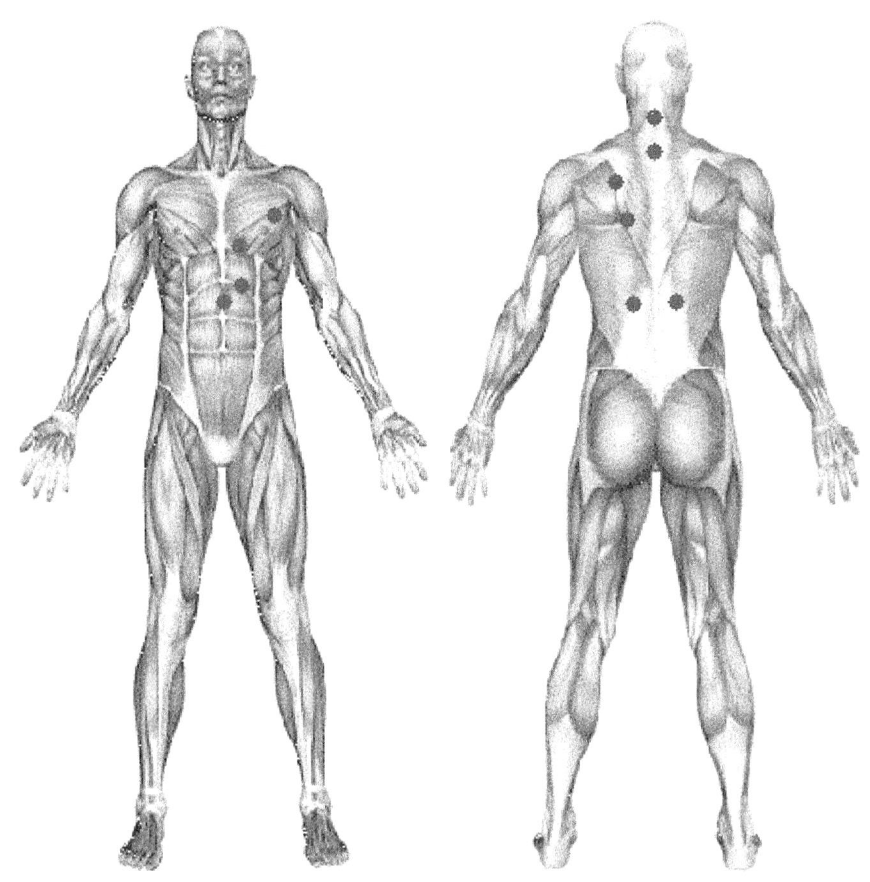

10 Cupping Points

10) Cupping for Elephantiasis

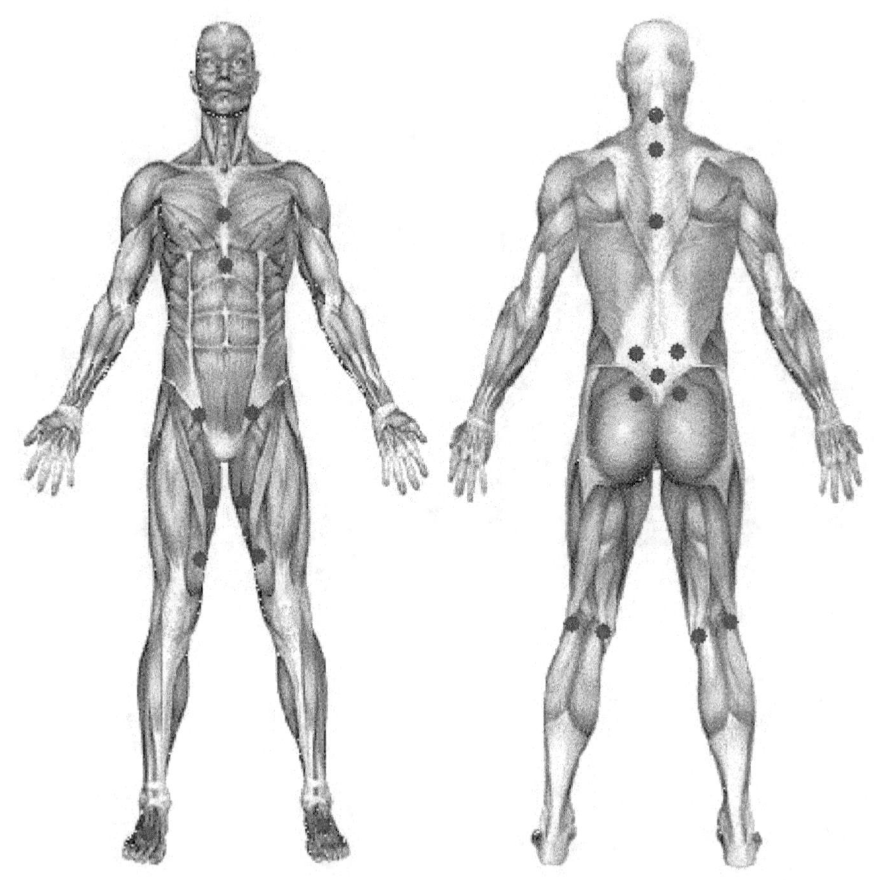

22 Cupping Points

11) Cupping for Asthma

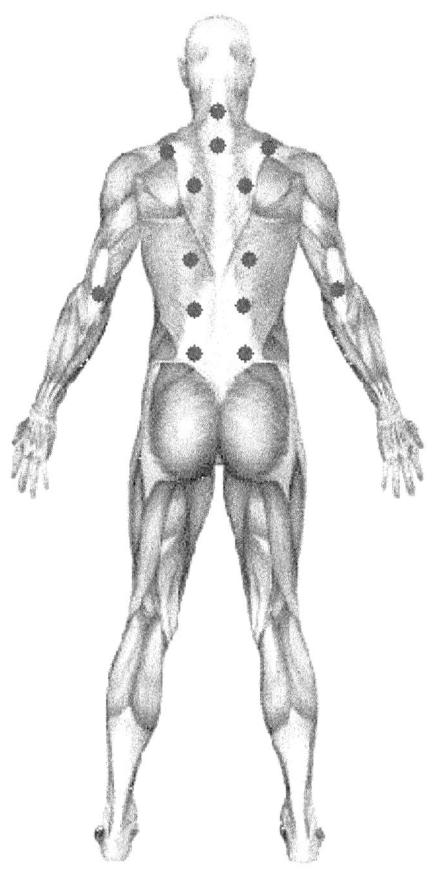

14 Cupping Points

12) Cupping for Insomnia (Difficulties to sleep at night)

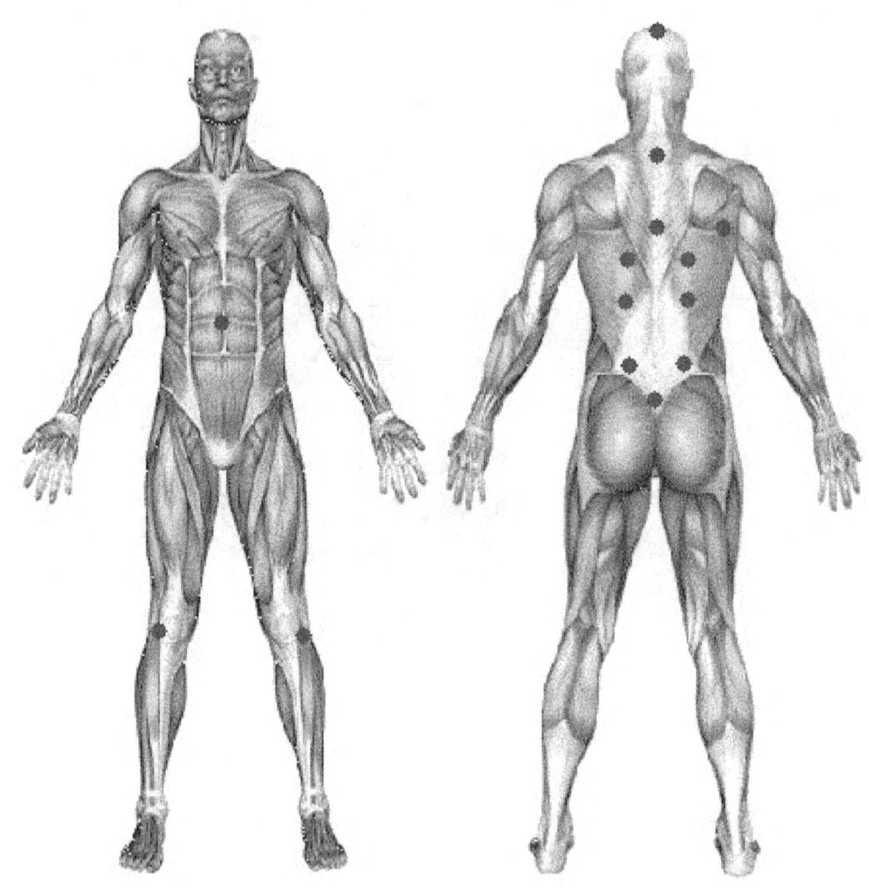

14 Cupping Points

13) Cupping for Diarrhoea

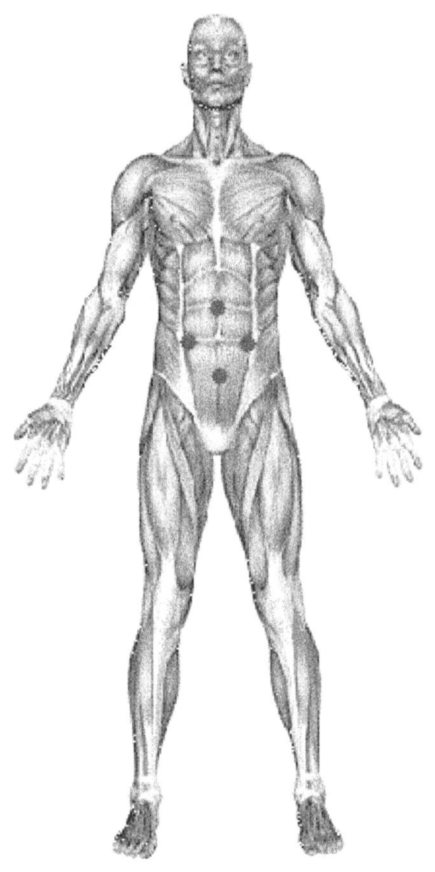

4 Cupping Points

14) Cupping for Muscle Cramps

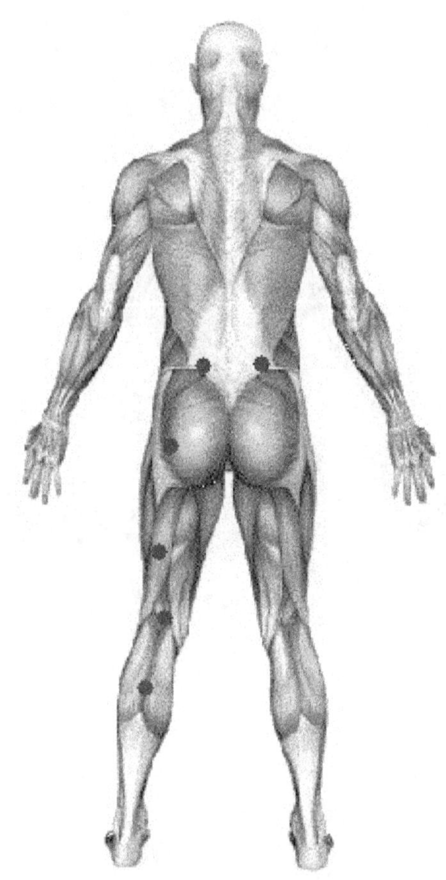

6 Cupping Points

15) Cupping for Decreasing Rib and Inflammatory Functions

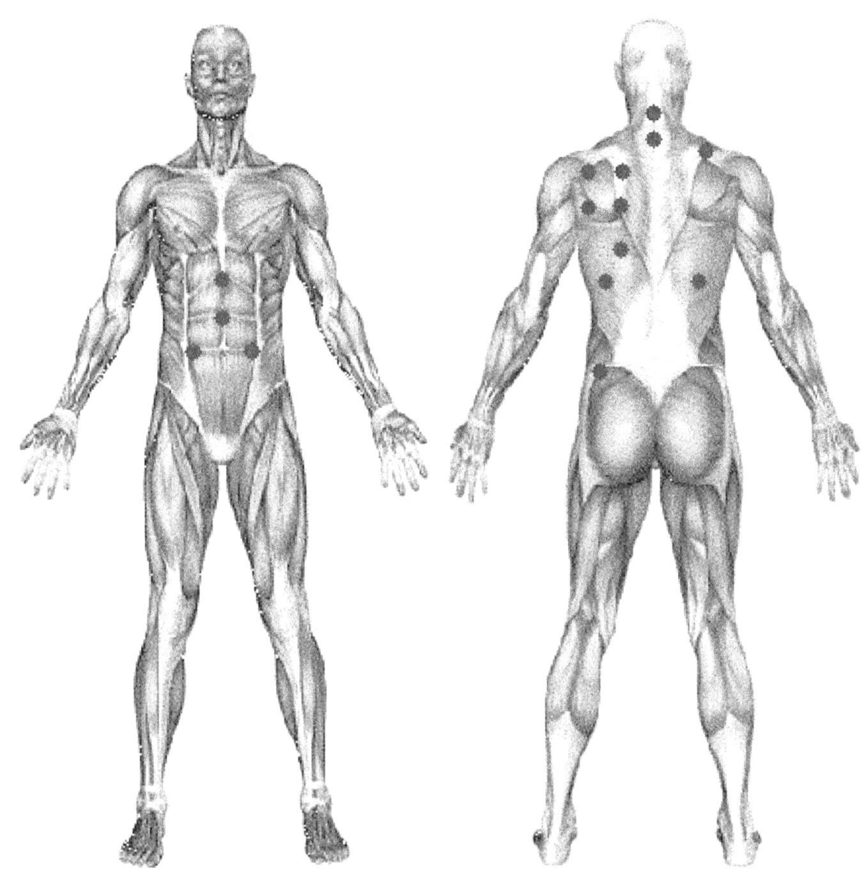

15 Cupping Points

16) Cupping for Food Allergy

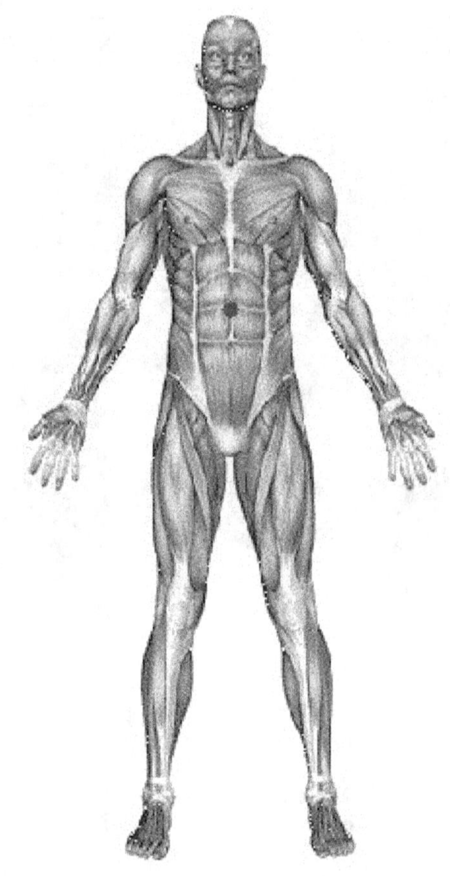

1 Cupping Point

17) Cupping for Bone Sore

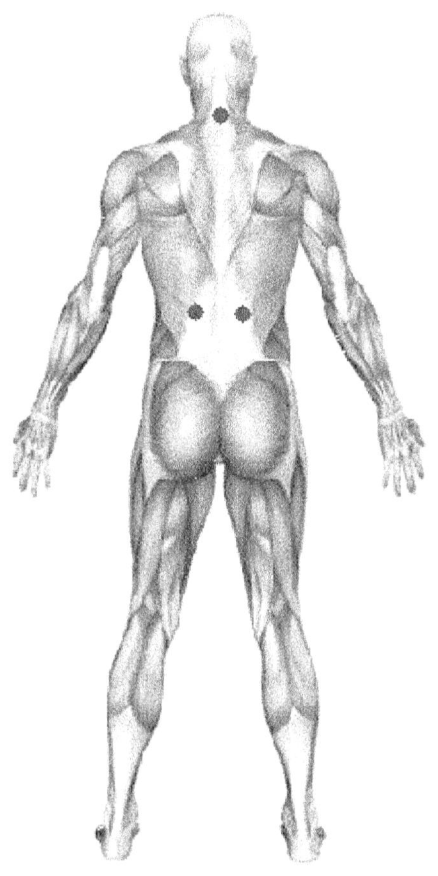

3 Cupping Points

18) Cupping for Breathing Difficulty

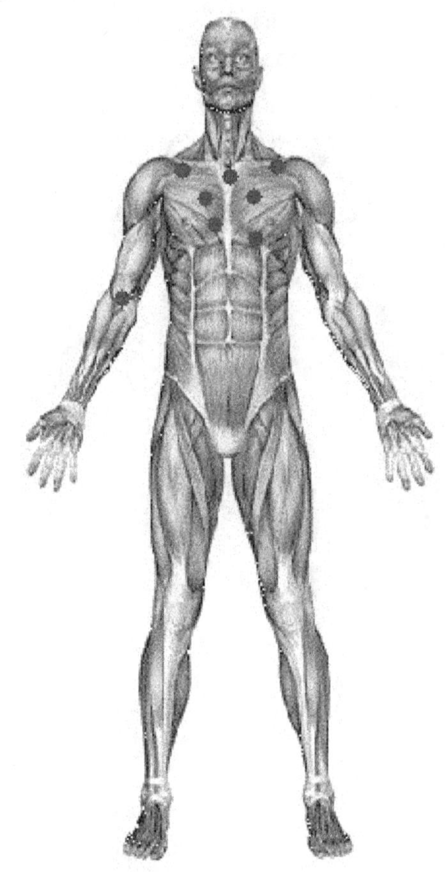

8 Cupping Points

19) Cupping for Bed-wetting

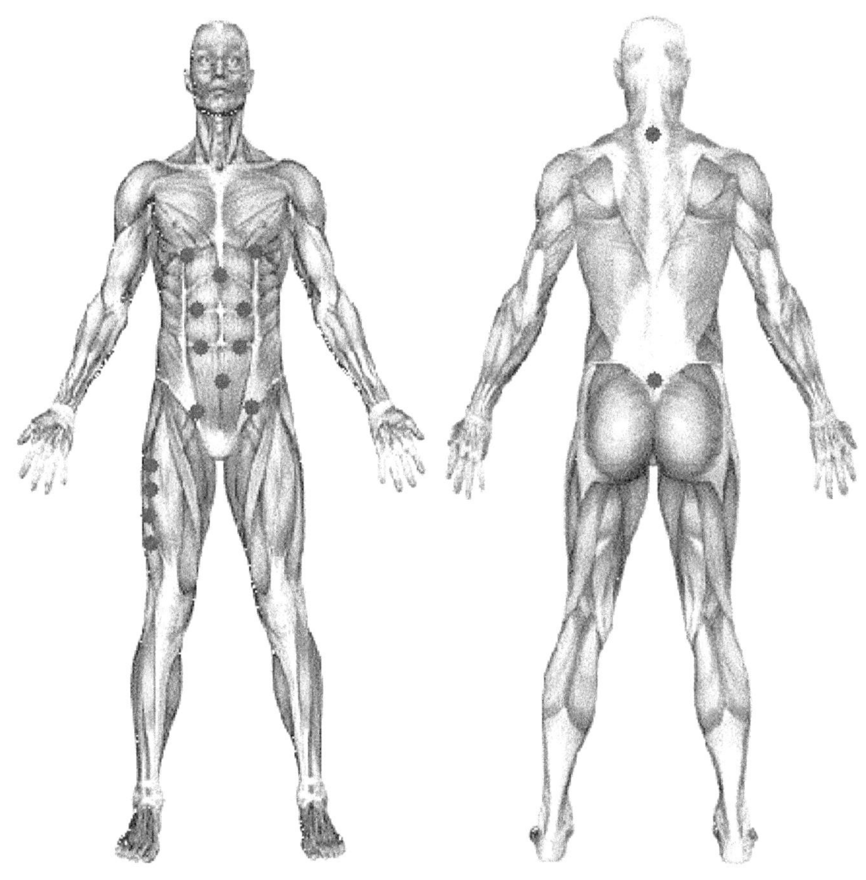

16 Cupping Points

20) Cupping for Tonsil

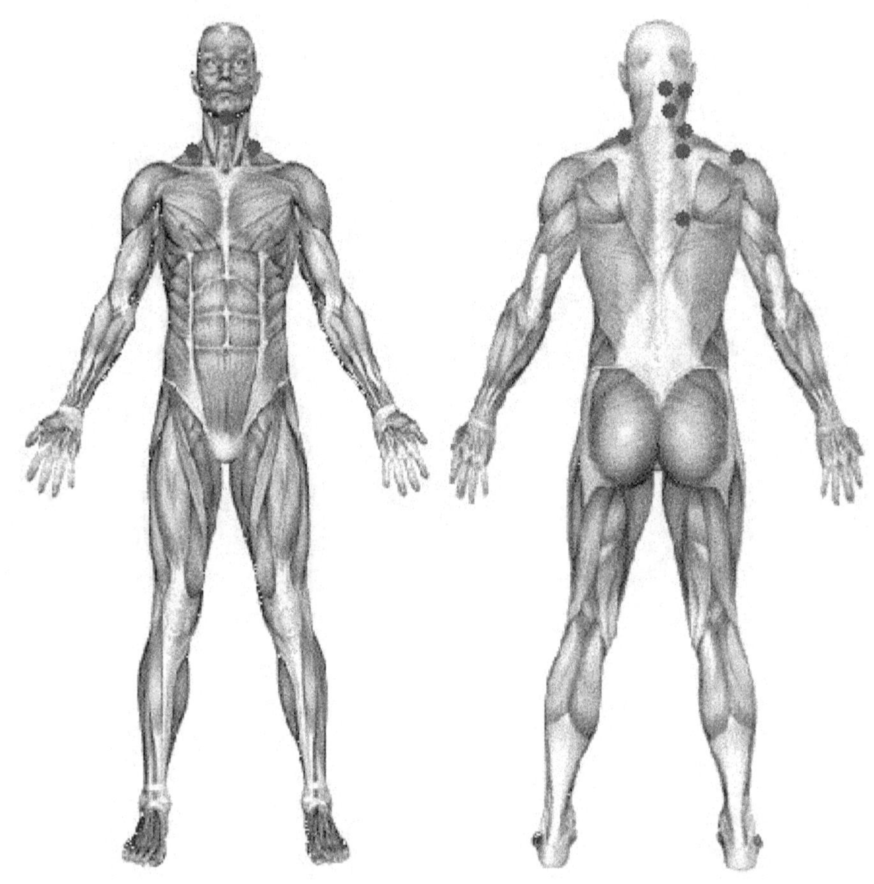

11 Cupping Points

21) Cupping for Itchiness

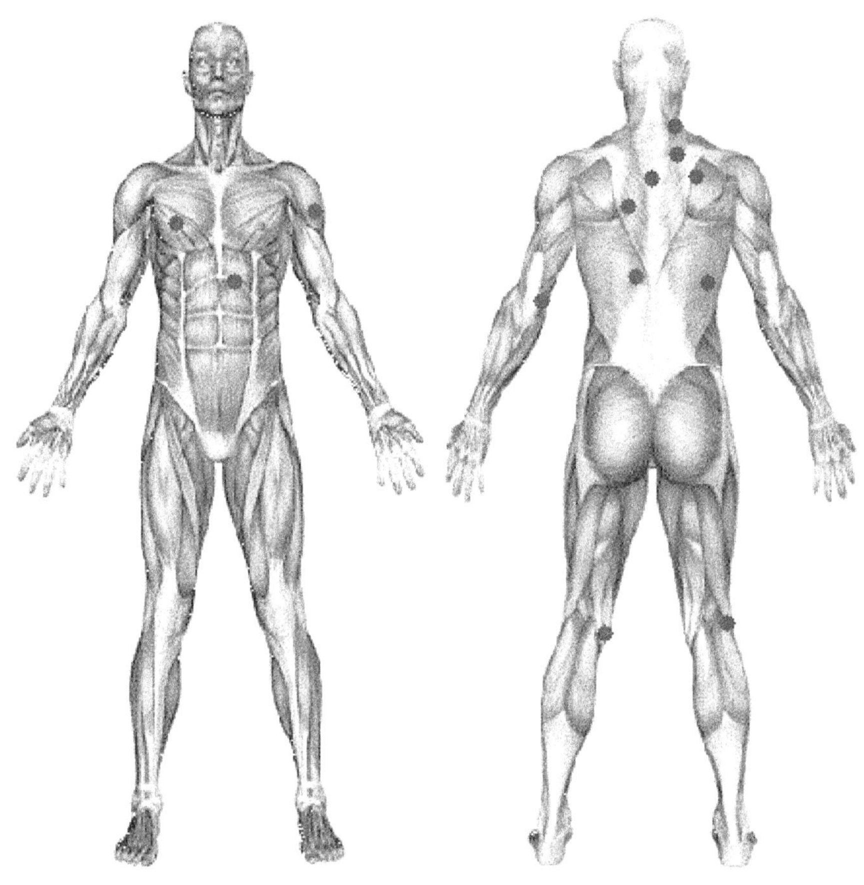

12 Cupping Points

22) Cupping for Diabetes

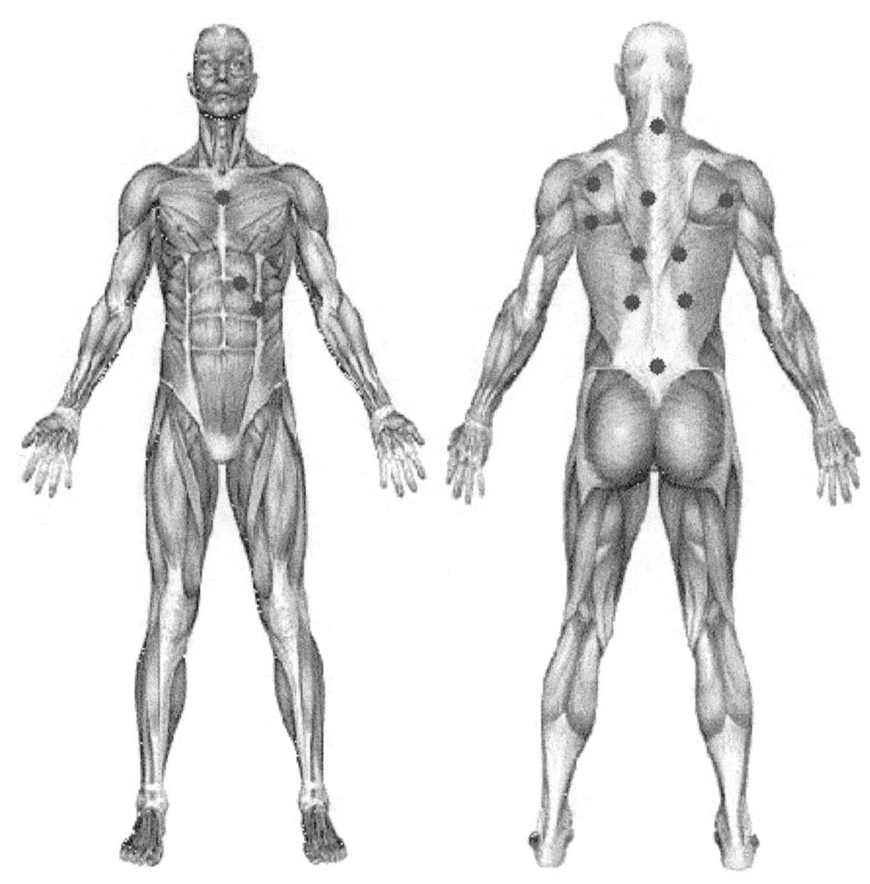

13 Cupping Points

23) Cupping for Gall Bladder and Liver Disorders

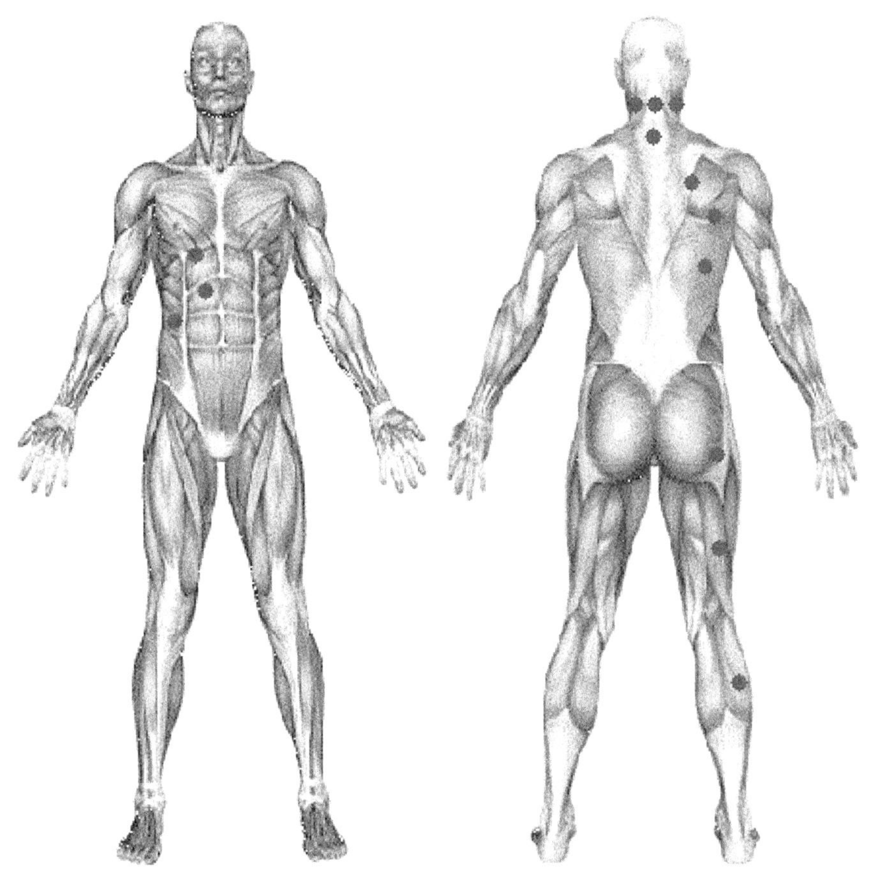

13 Cupping Points

24) Cupping for Shivering without Fever

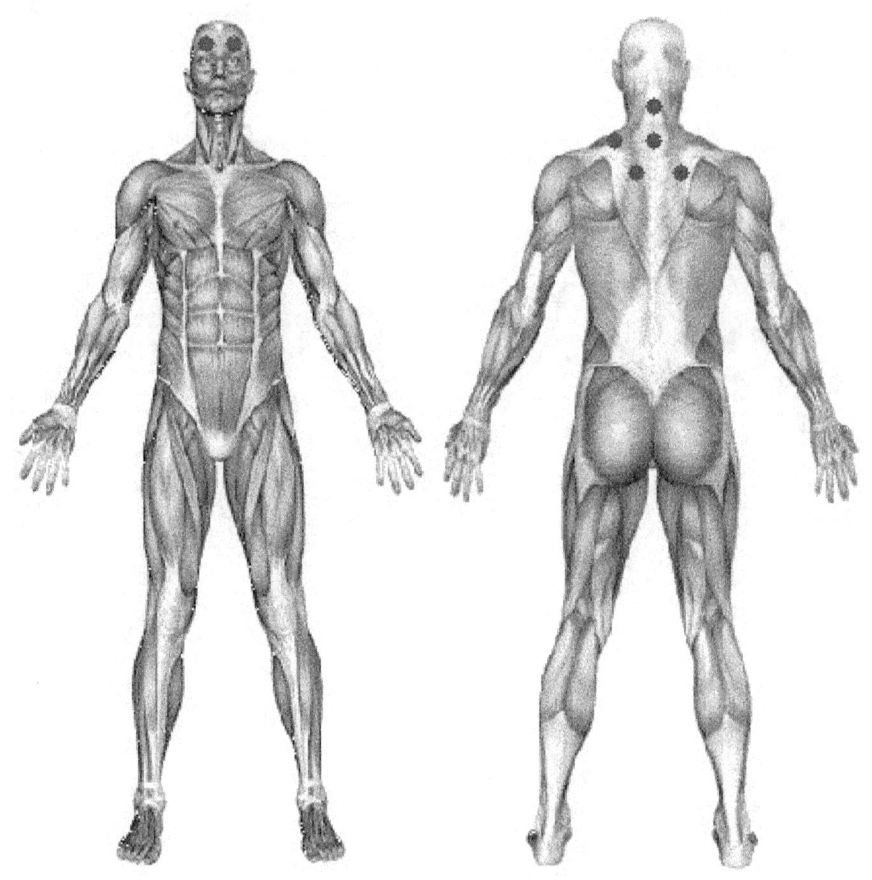

7 Cupping Points

25) Cupping for Irregular Period

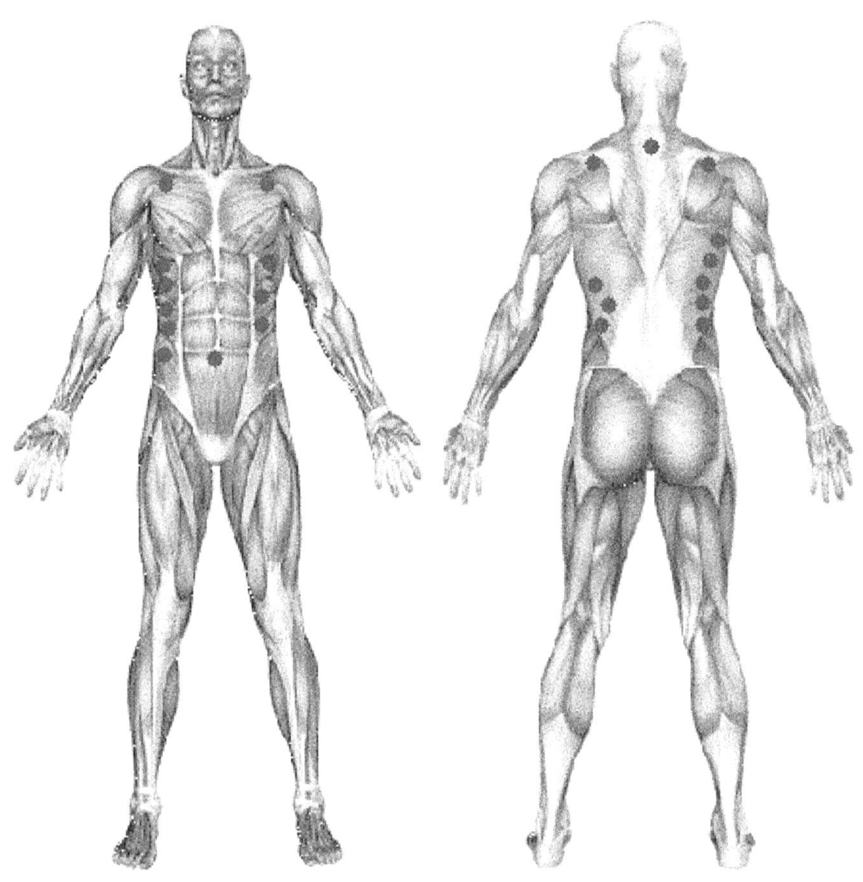

22 Cupping Points

26) Cupping for Kidney

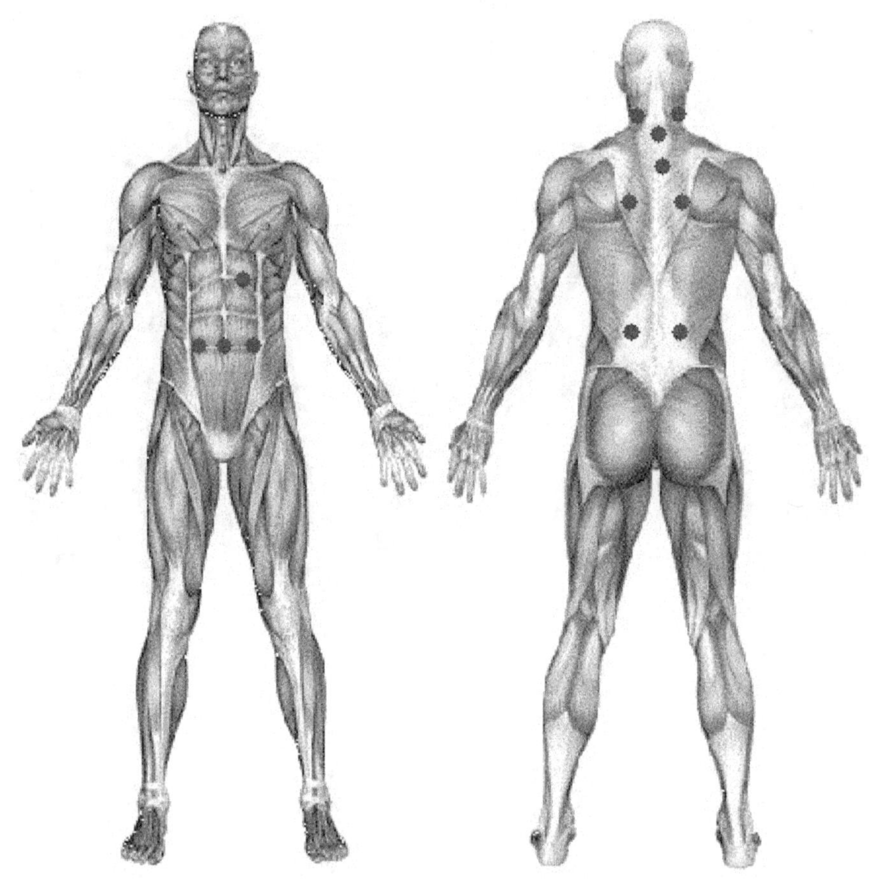

12 Cupping Points

27) Cupping for Hypertension

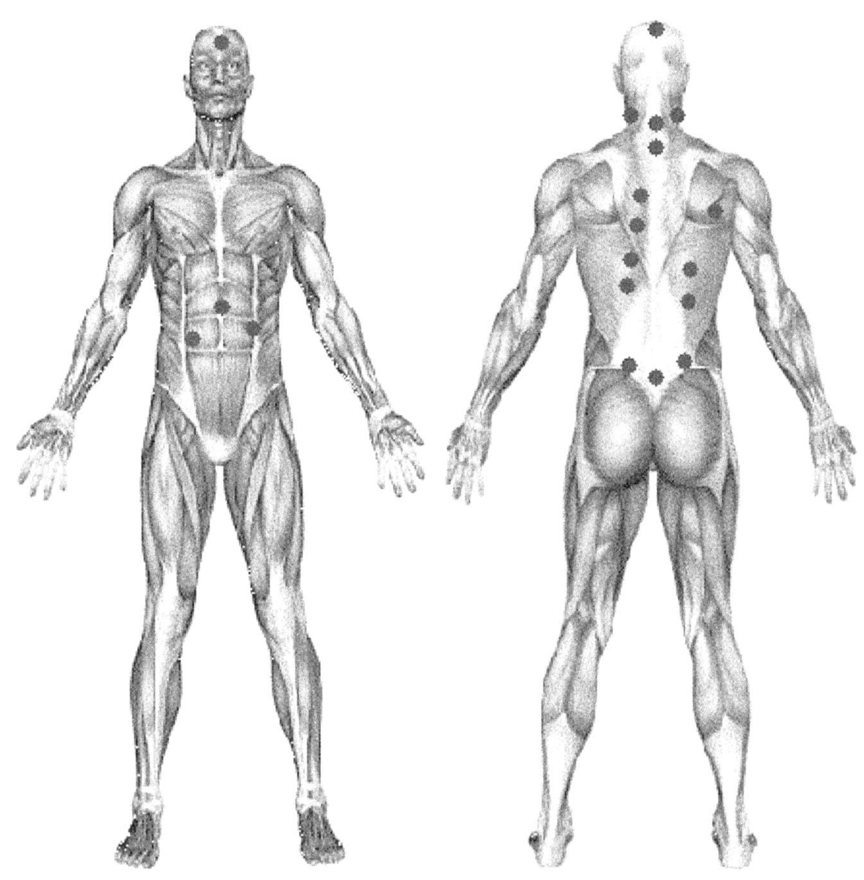

19 Cupping Points

28) Cupping for Colon Inflammation

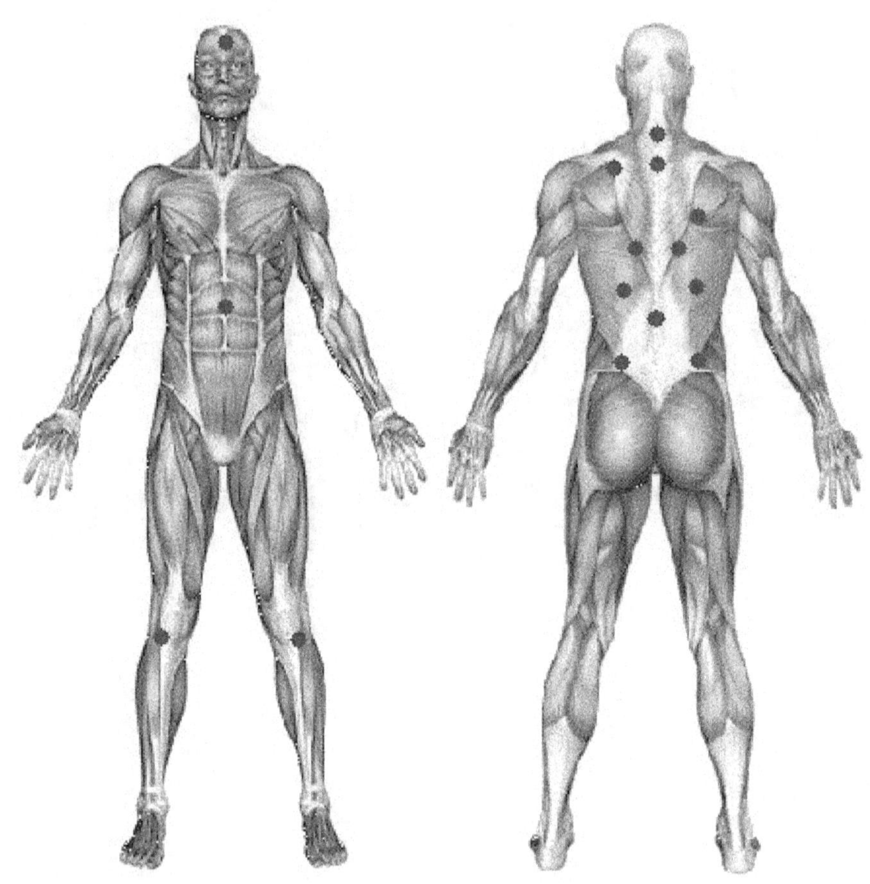

14 Cupping Points

29) Cupping for Heavy Depression

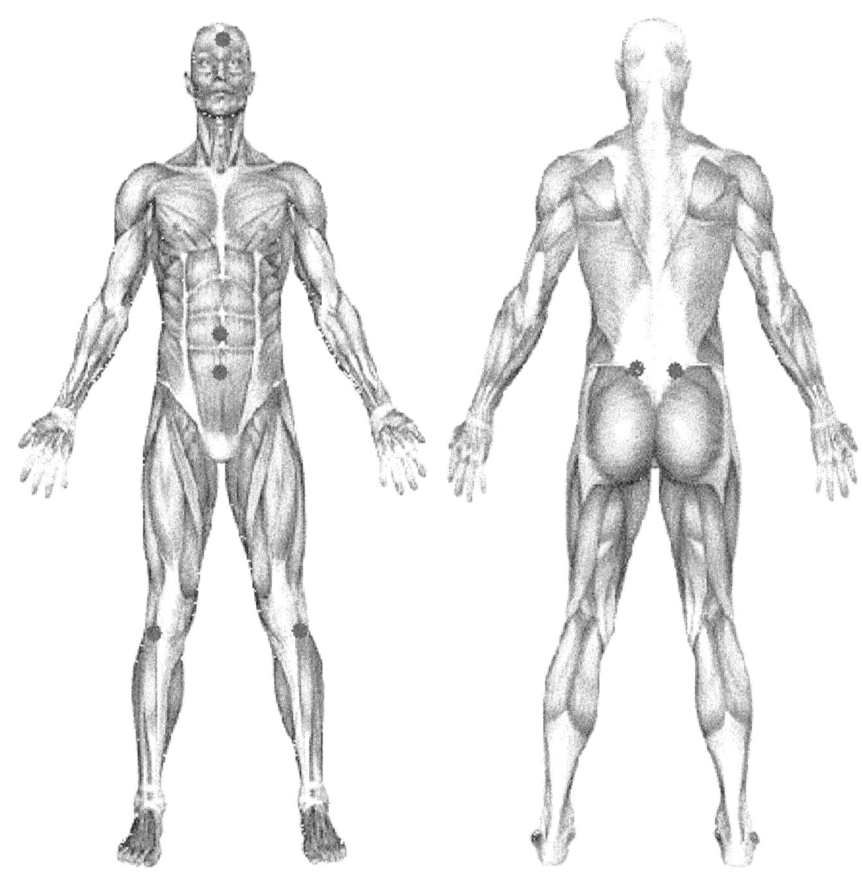

6 Cupping Points

30) Cupping for Bladder Disorder

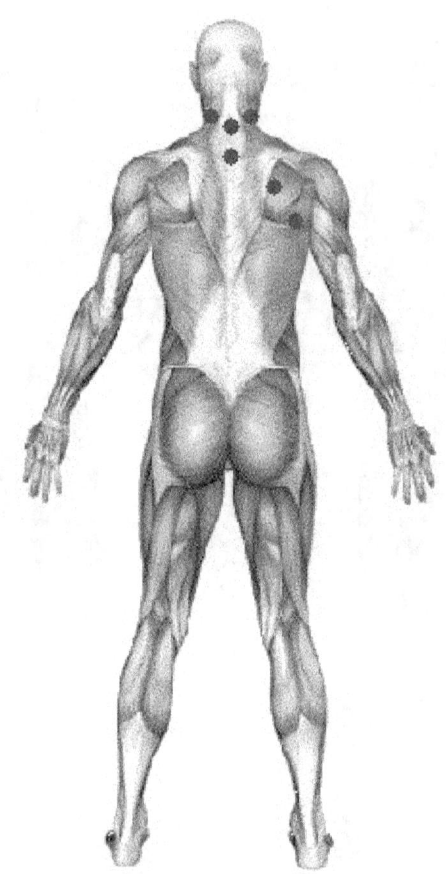

6 Cupping Points

31) Cupping for Stroke

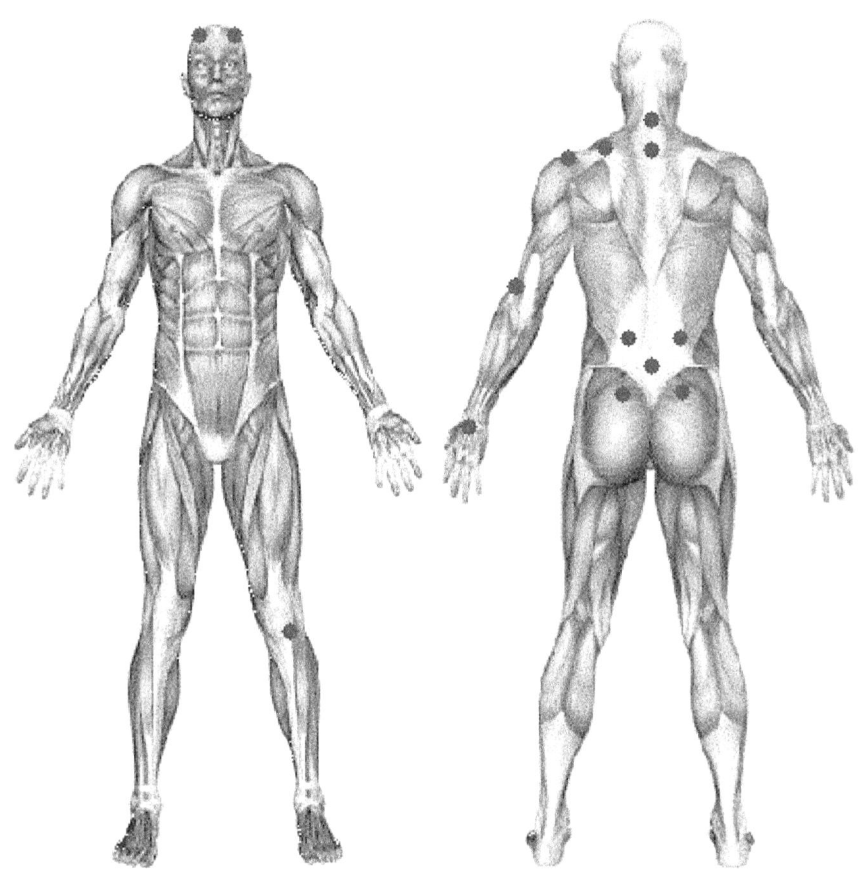

14 Cupping Points

32) Cupping for Gout

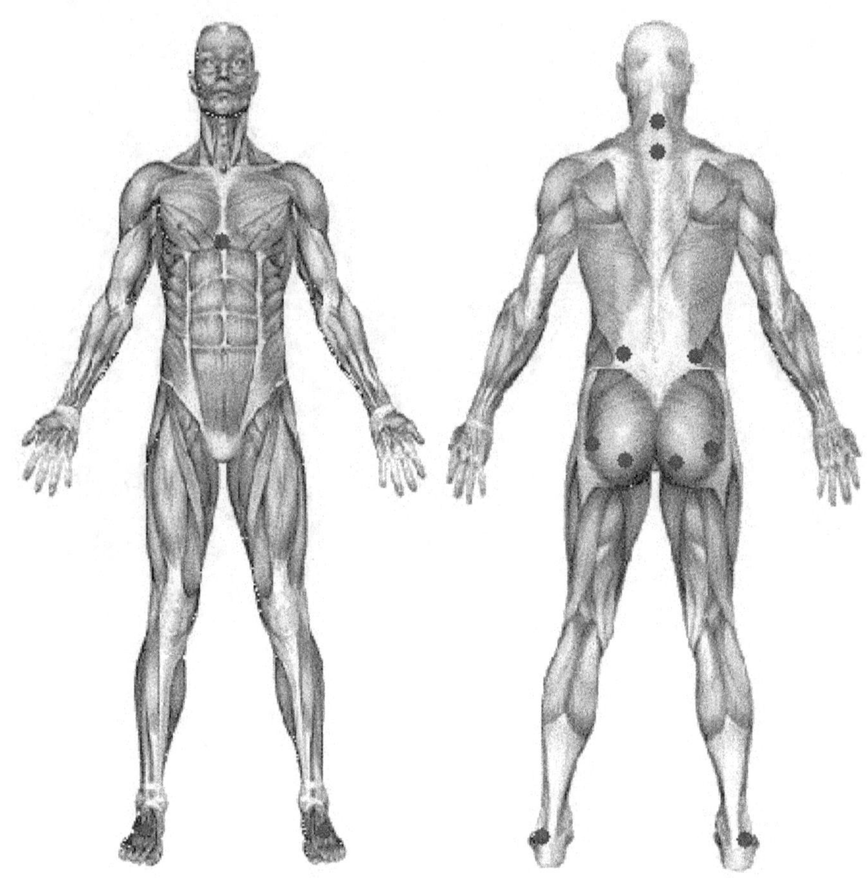

13 Cupping Points

33) Cupping for Rheumatoid

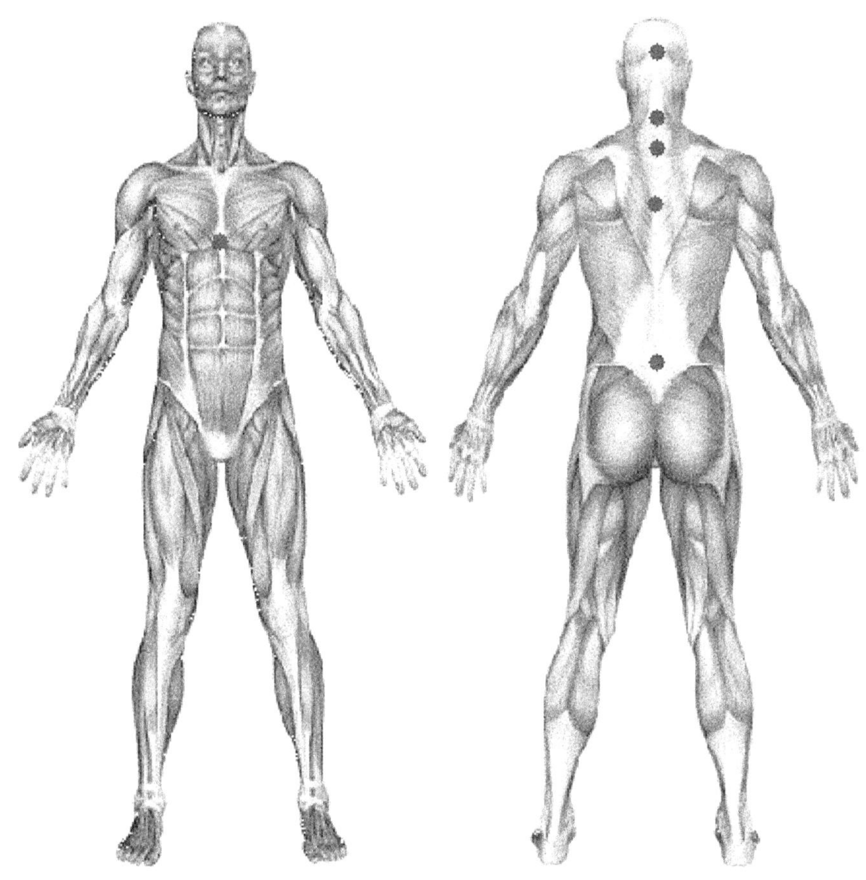

6 Cupping Points

34) Cupping for Knee Pain

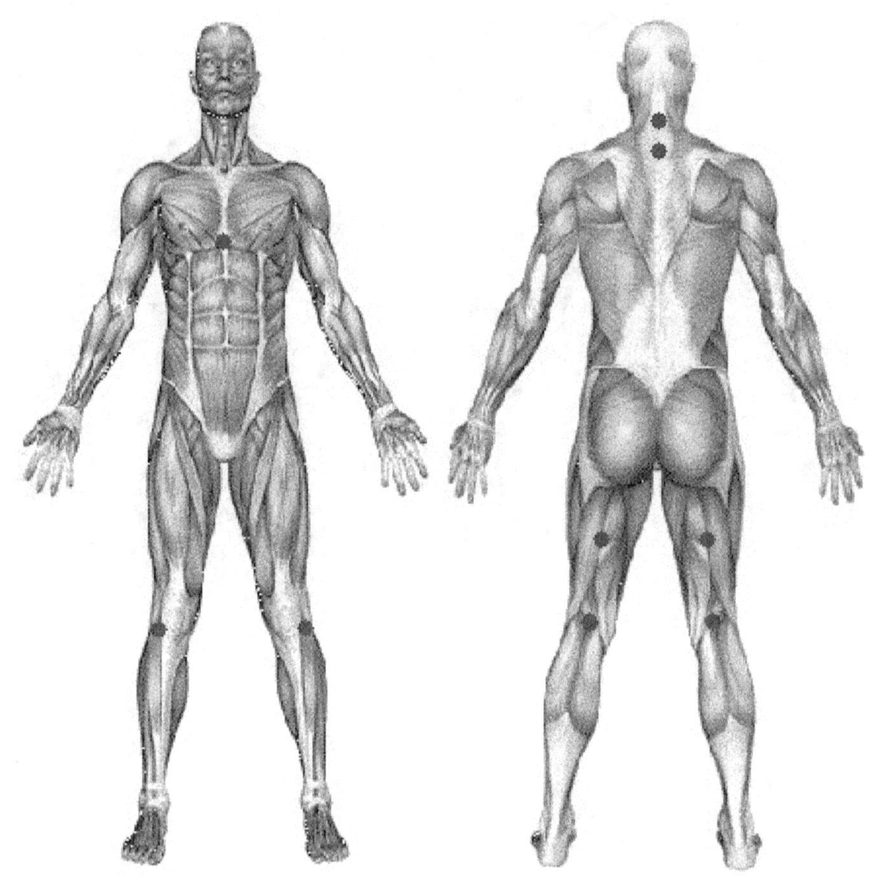

9 Cupping Points

35) Cupping for Pain in the Legs

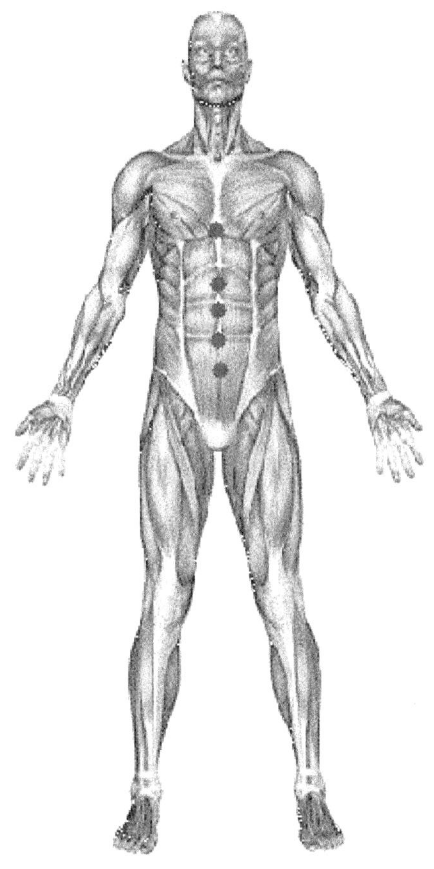

5 Cupping Points

36) Cupping for Pain around the Spine

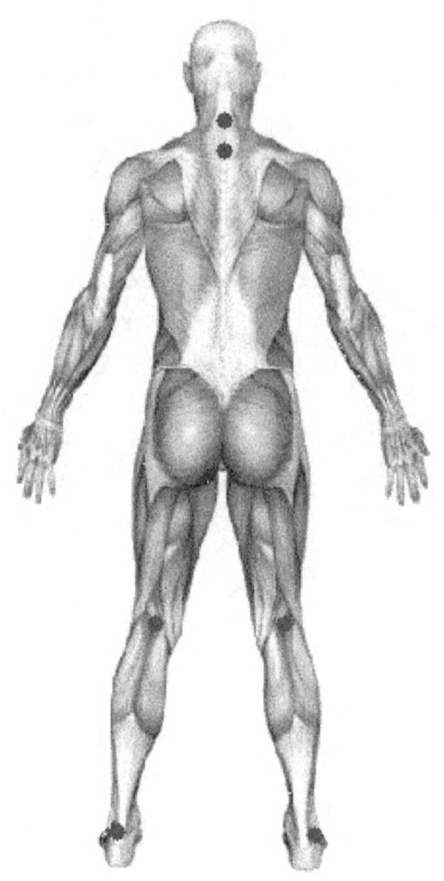

6 Cupping Points

37) Cupping for Mental Disorder

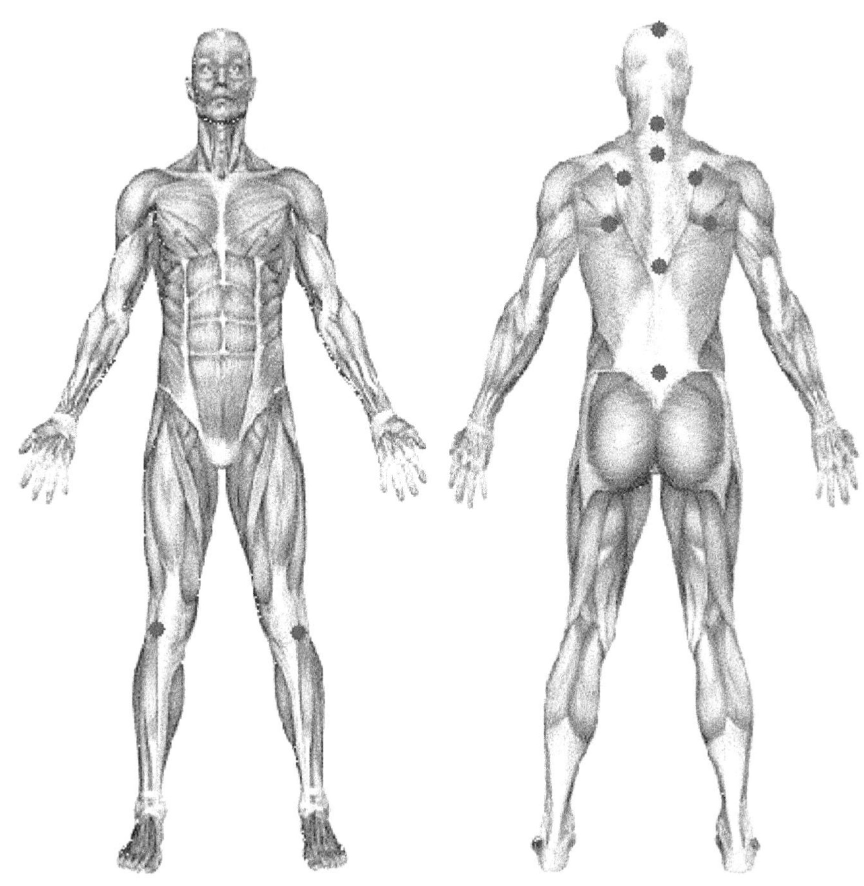

11 Cupping Points

38) Cupping for Pain in the Stomach Area

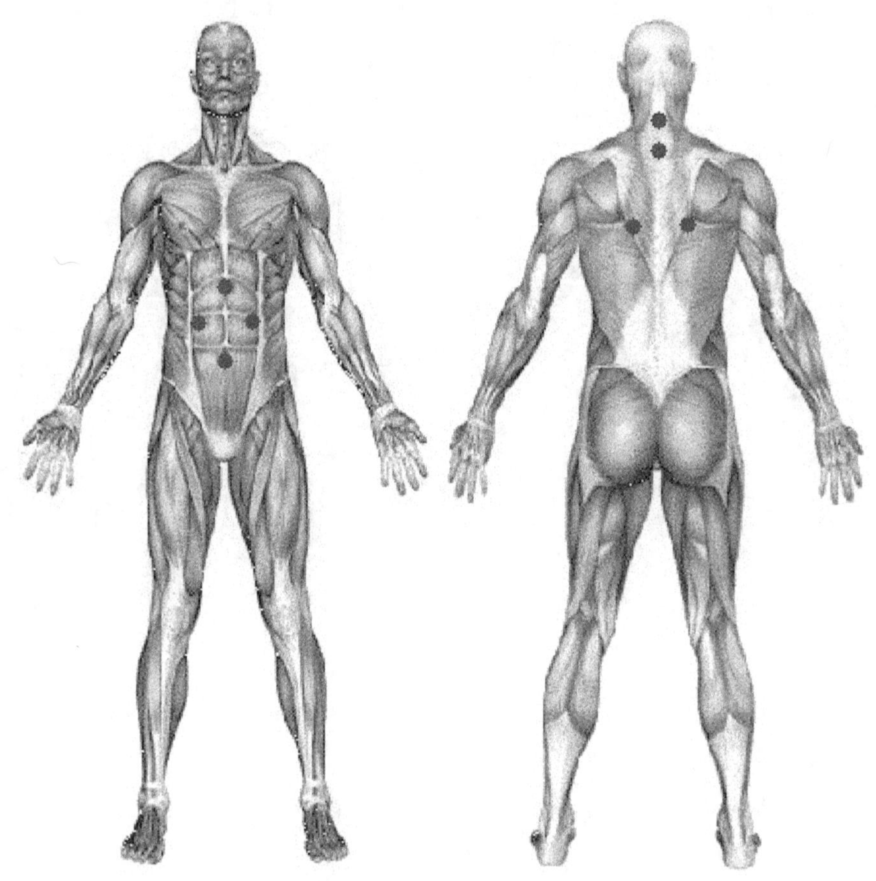

8 Cupping Points

39) Cupping for Rib Disorder and Rib Skin Disease

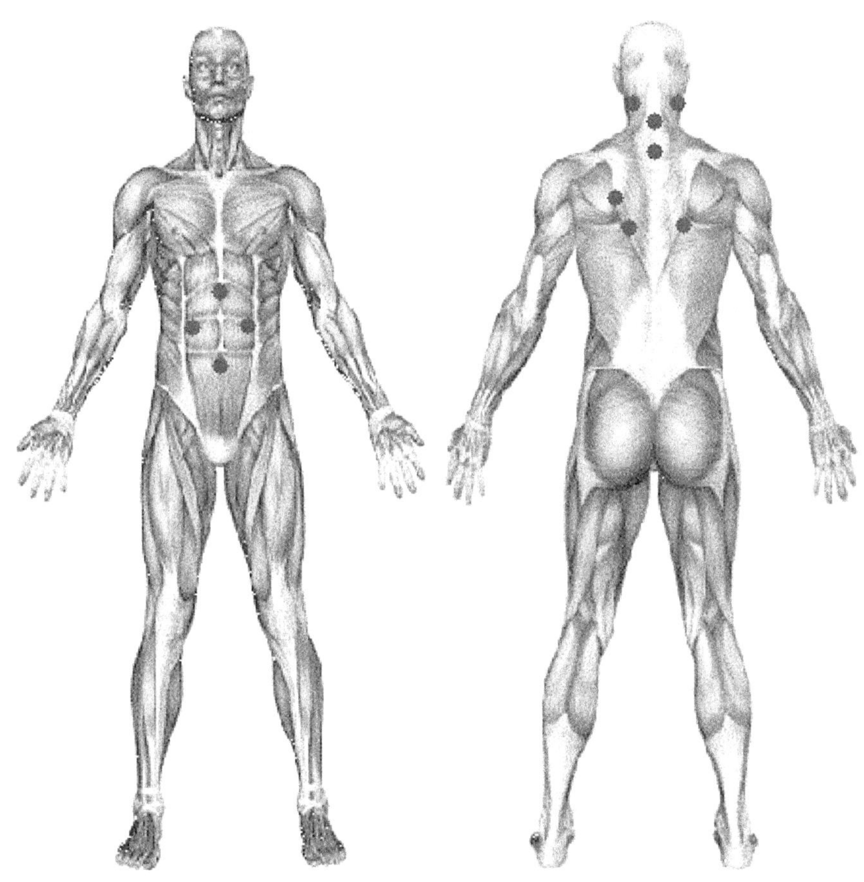

11 Cupping Points

40) Cupping for Haemorrhoids

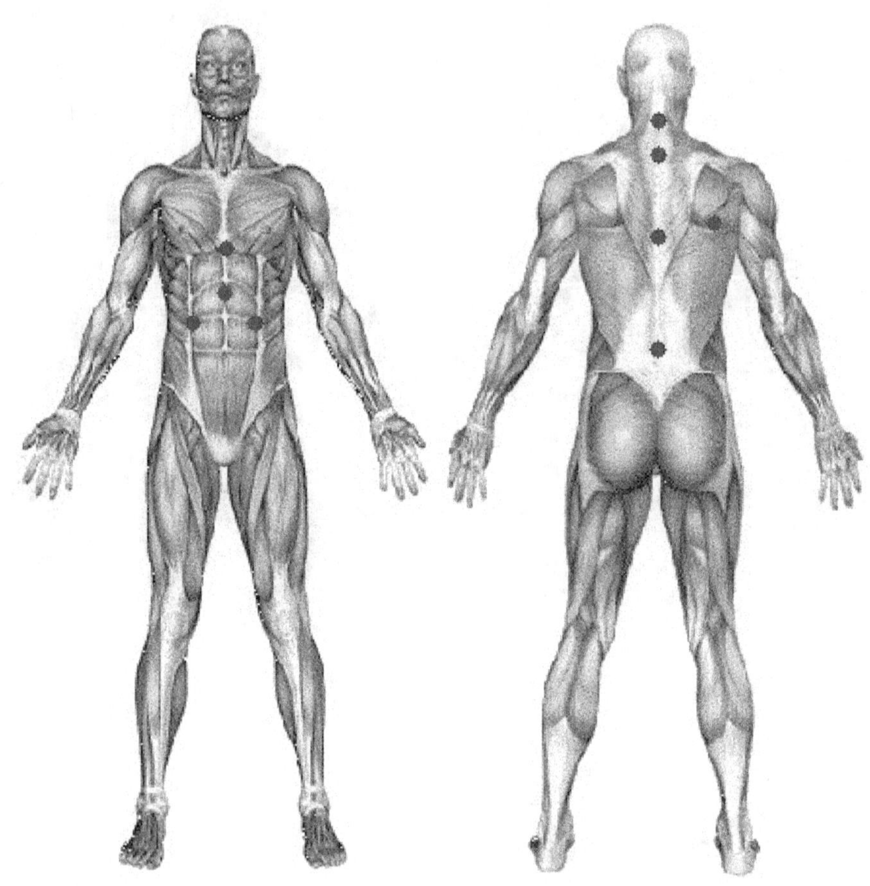

9 Cupping Points

41) Cupping for Wounds, Boils on the Calf and Buttocks and Itchiness

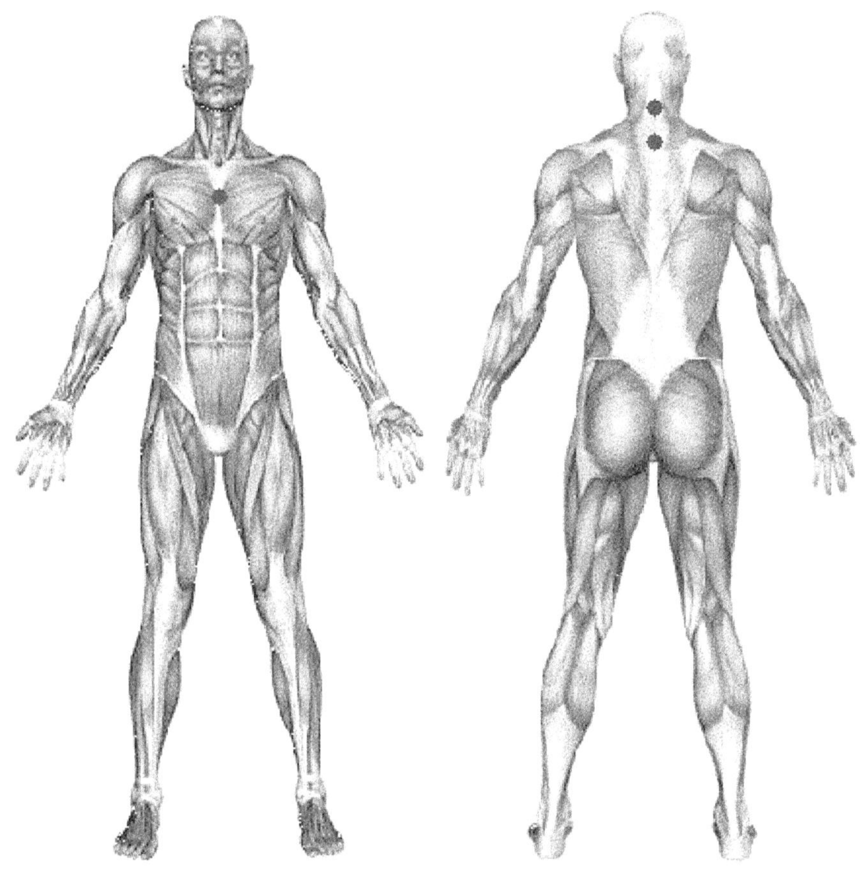

3 Cupping Points

42) Cupping for Decreased Body Endurance

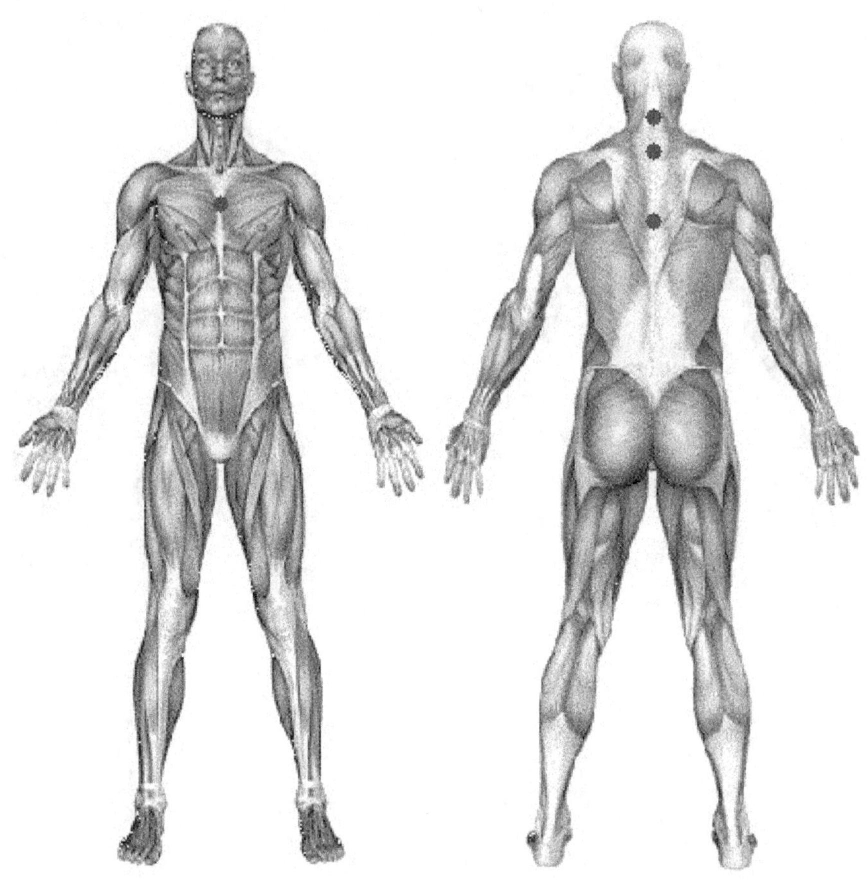

4 Cupping Points

43) Cupping for Sinus

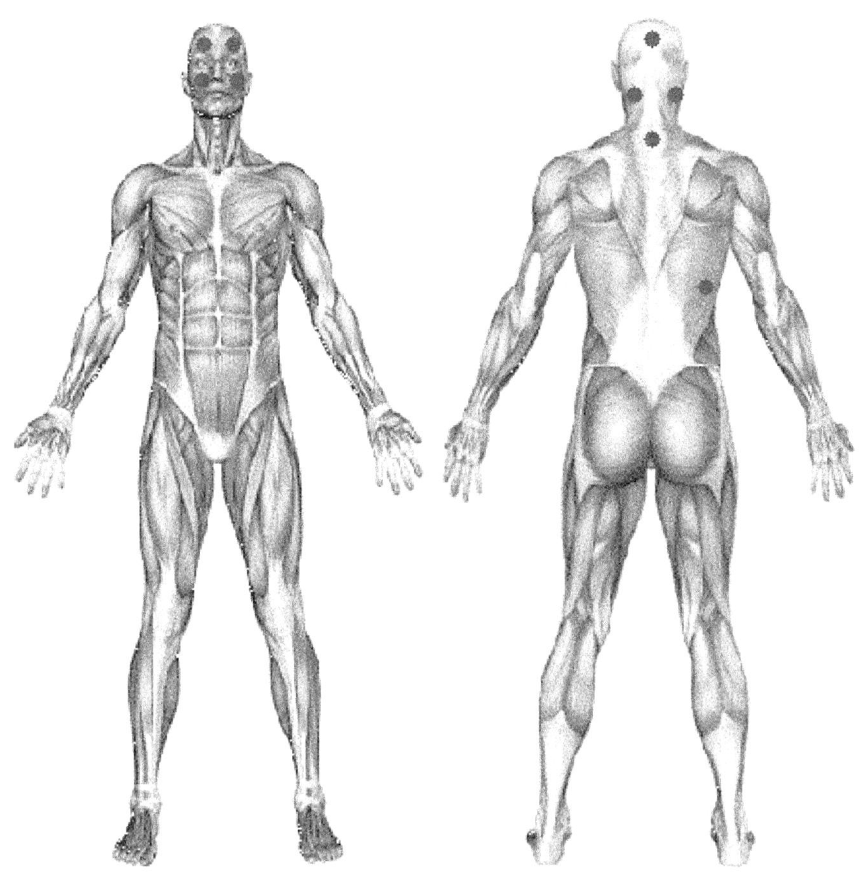

9 Cupping Points

44) Cupping for Improving Blood Circulation

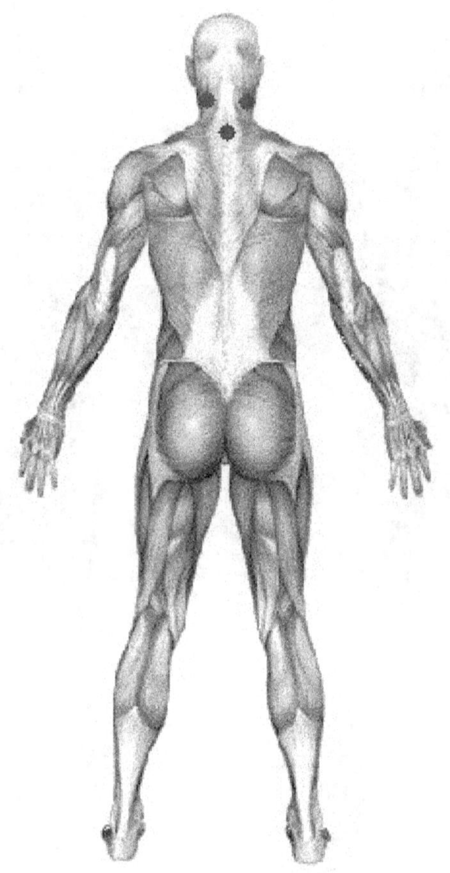

3 Cupping Points

45) Cupping for Narrow and Clogged Blood Vessels

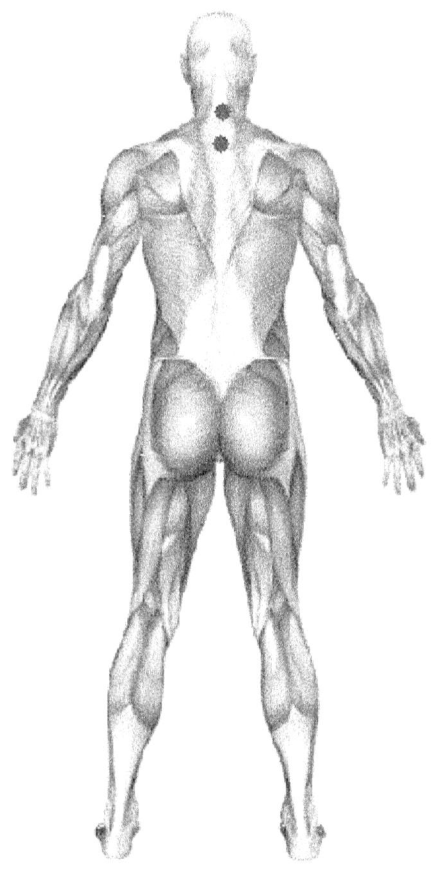

2 Cupping Points

46) Cupping for Sore Buttocks

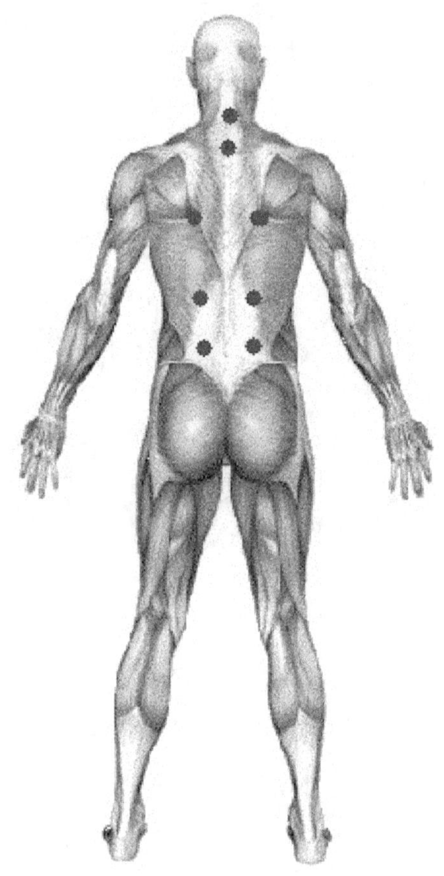

8 Waist Points

47) Cupping for Shoulder and Neck Pain

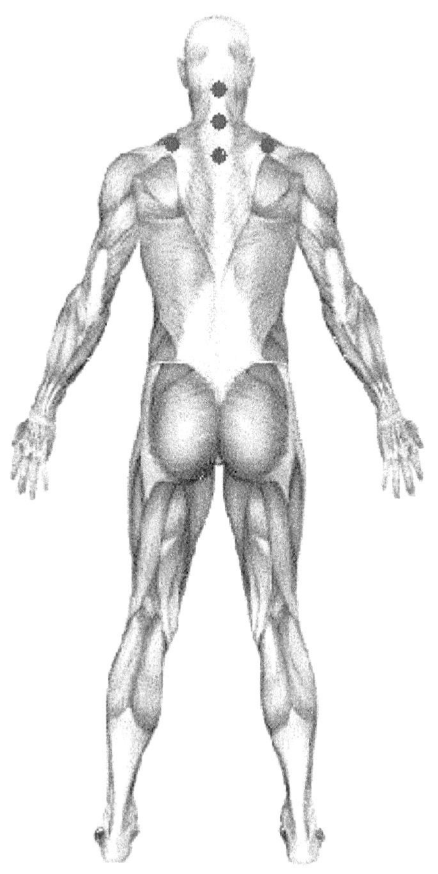

5 Cupping Points

48) Cupping for Headache and Drowsiness due to High Blood Pressure

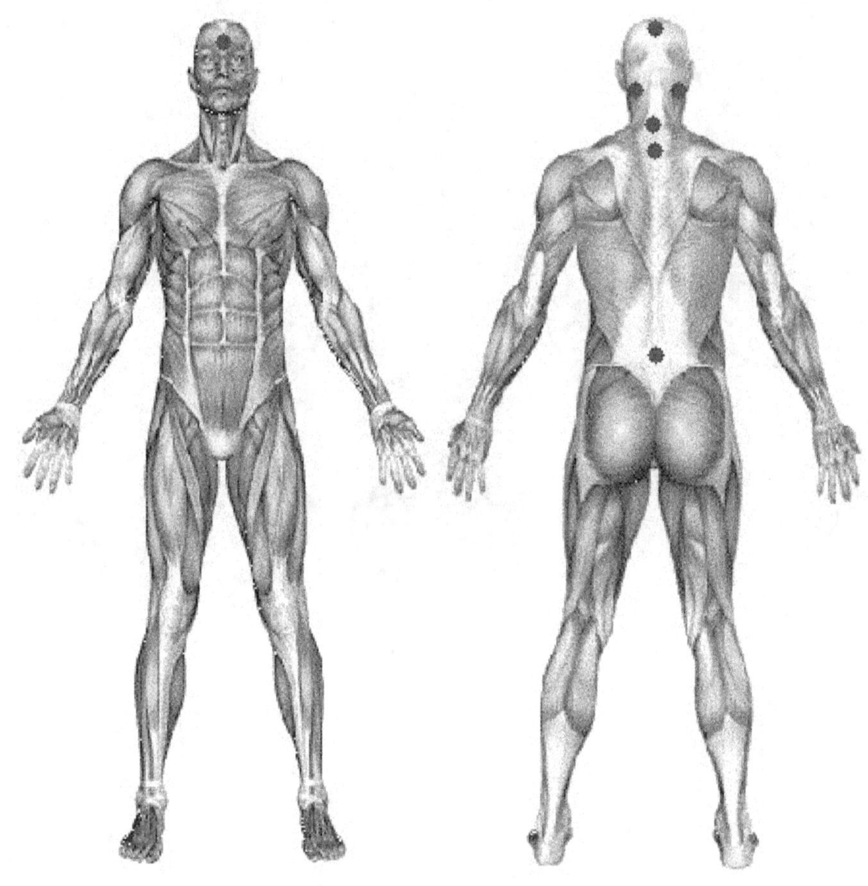

7 Cupping Points

49) Cupping for Heart Disease

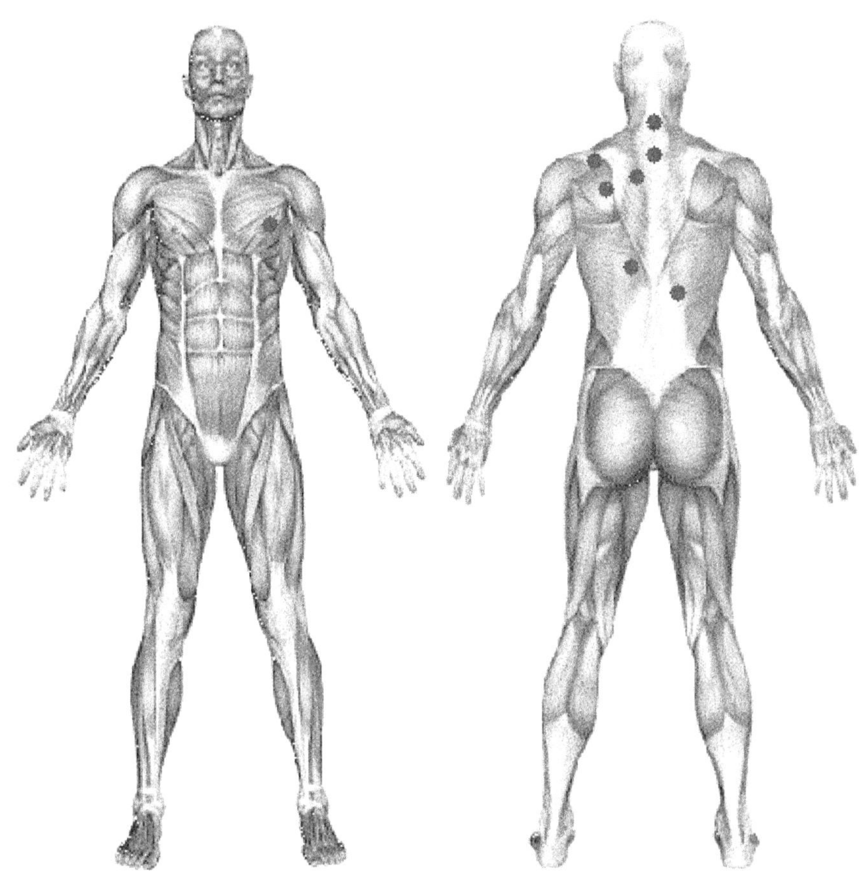

8 Cupping Points

50) Cupping for Infertility

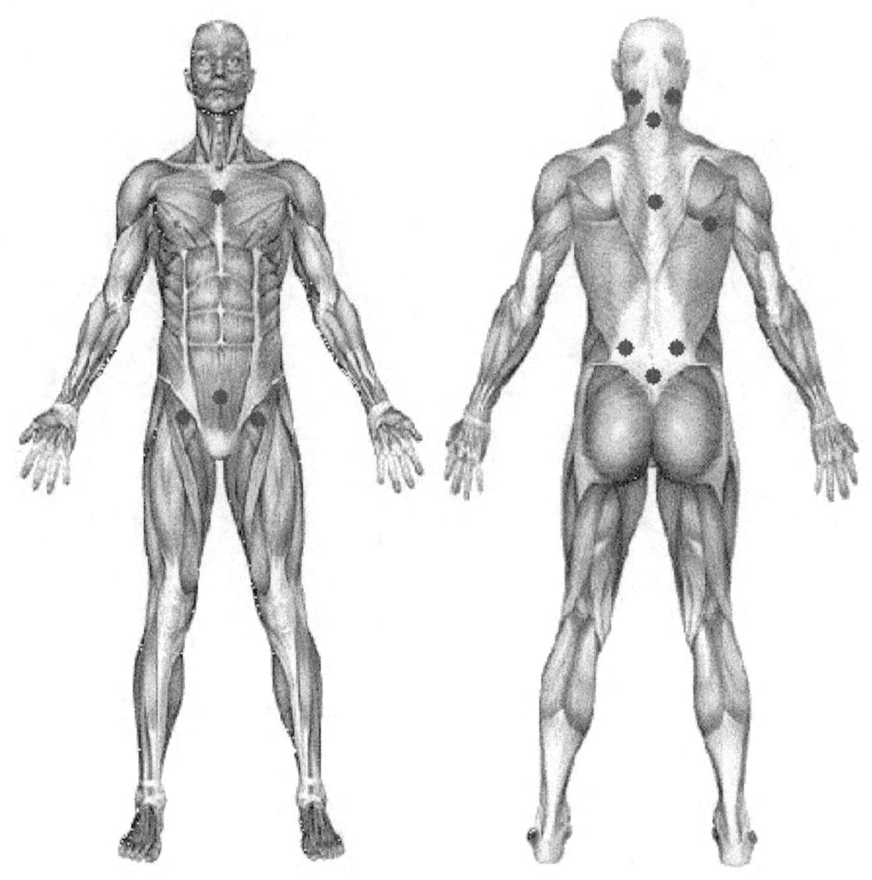

12 Cupping Points

51) Cupping for Excessive Sleeping

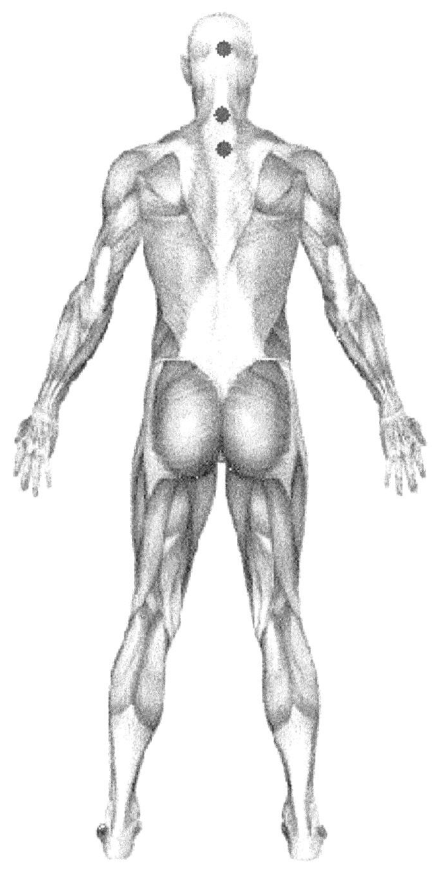

3 Cupping Points

52) Cupping for Migraine

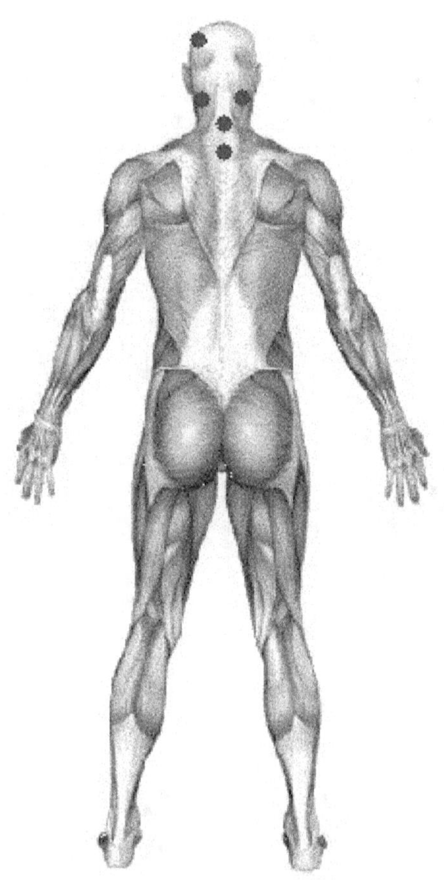

5 Cupping Points

53) Cupping for Decreased Blood Flow

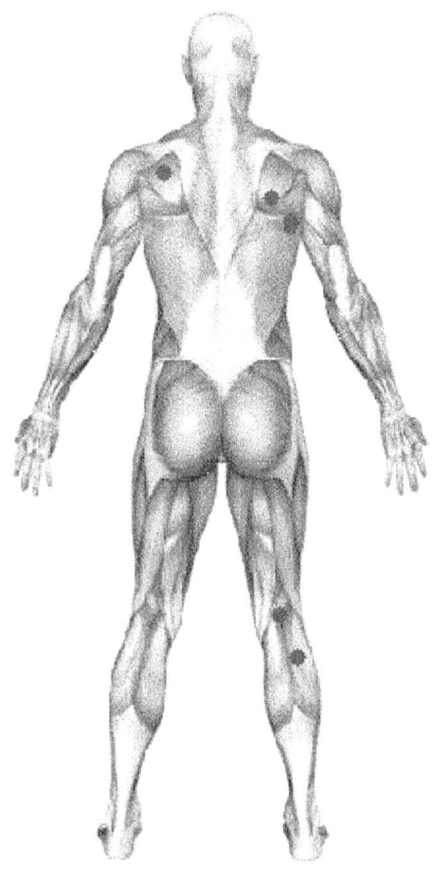

5 Cupping Points

54) Cupping for Improving Memory

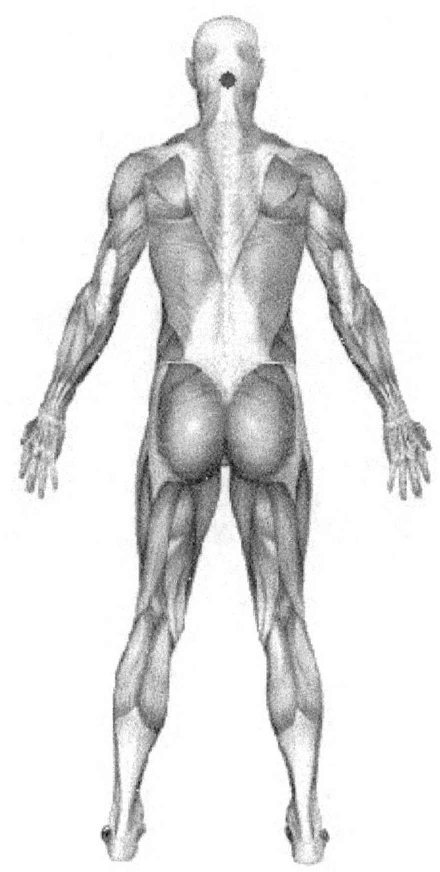

1 Cupping Point

55) Cupping for Improving Concentration

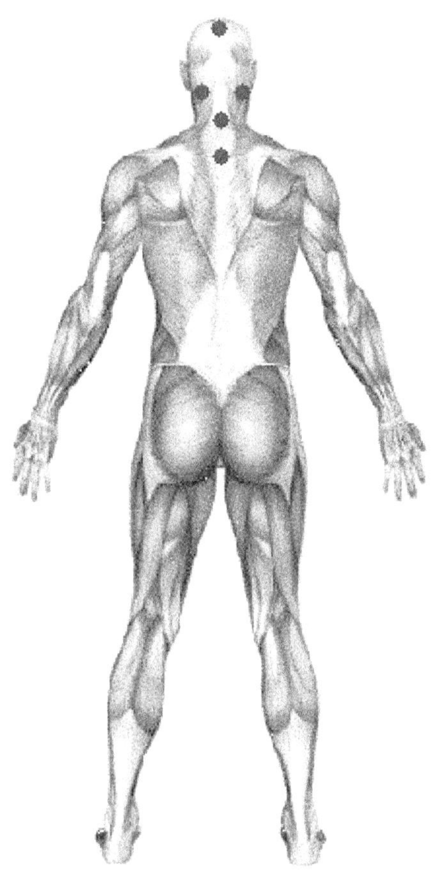

5 Cupping Points

56) Cupping for Anal Fistula

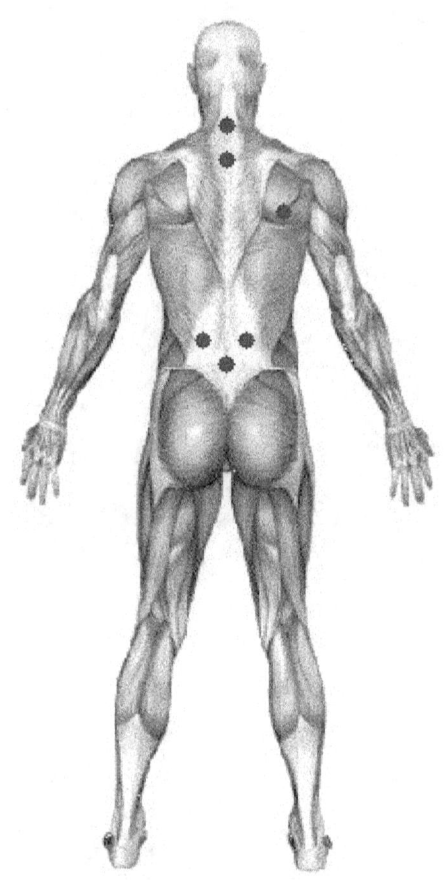

6 Cupping Points

57) Cupping for Bladder Disorder

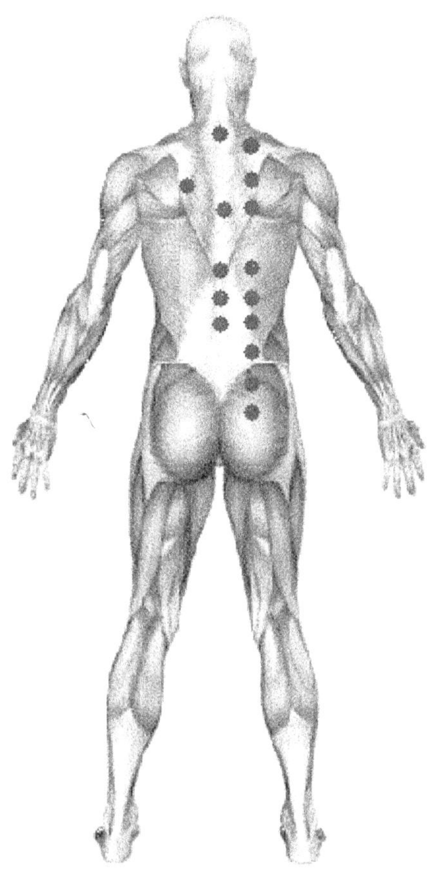

15 Cupping Points

58) Cupping for Skinny Body

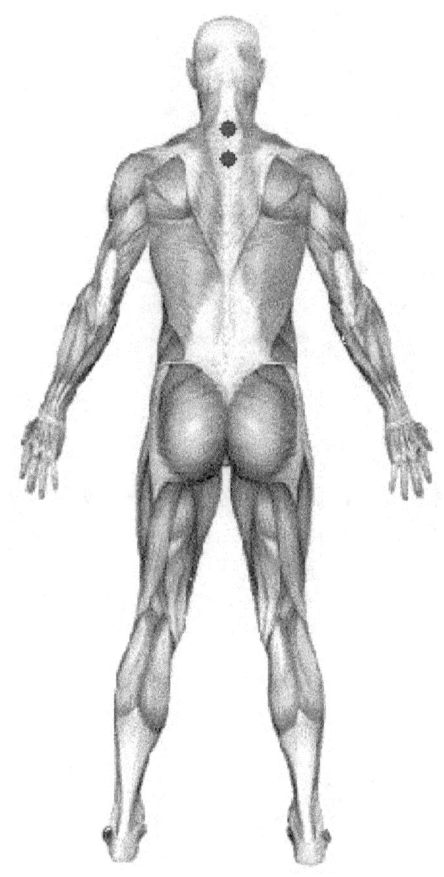

2 Cupping Points

59) Cupping for Quitting Smoking

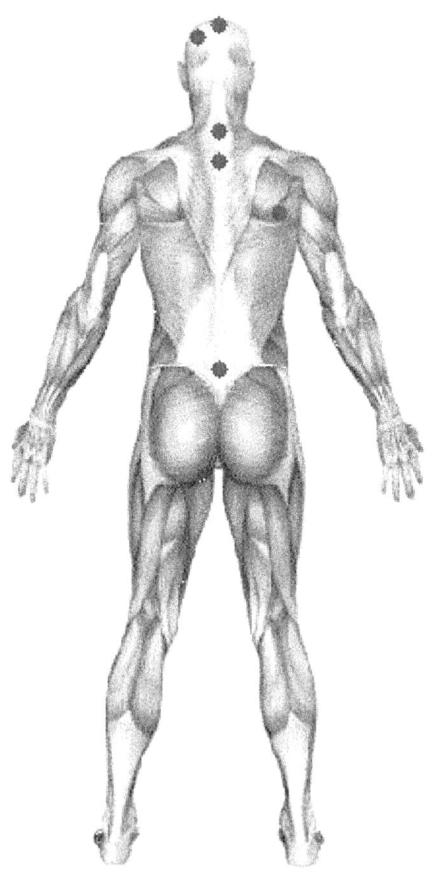

6 Cupping Points

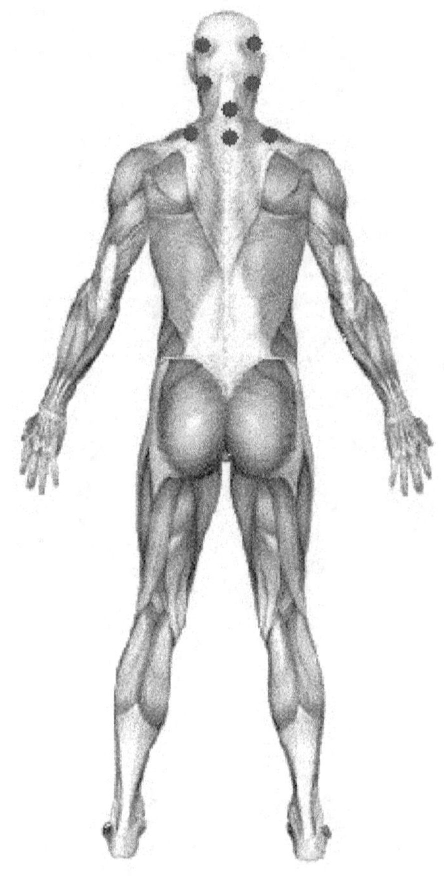

6 Cupping Points

61) Cupping for Germ Infection

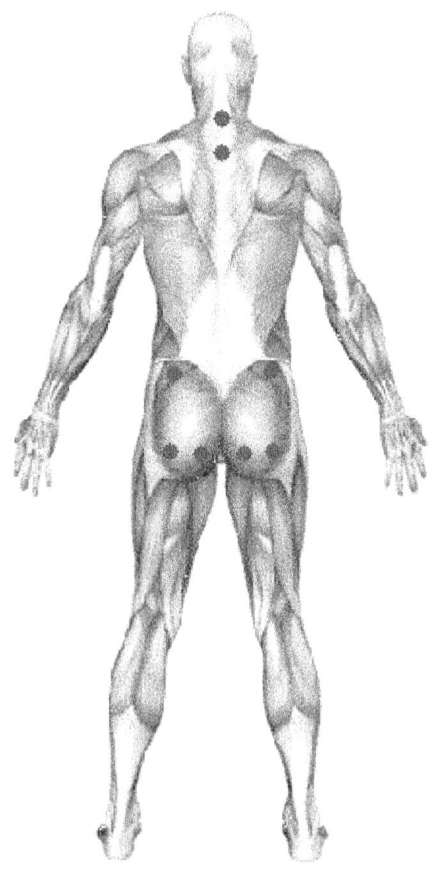

8 Cupping Points

62) Cupping for Improving Blood Circulation

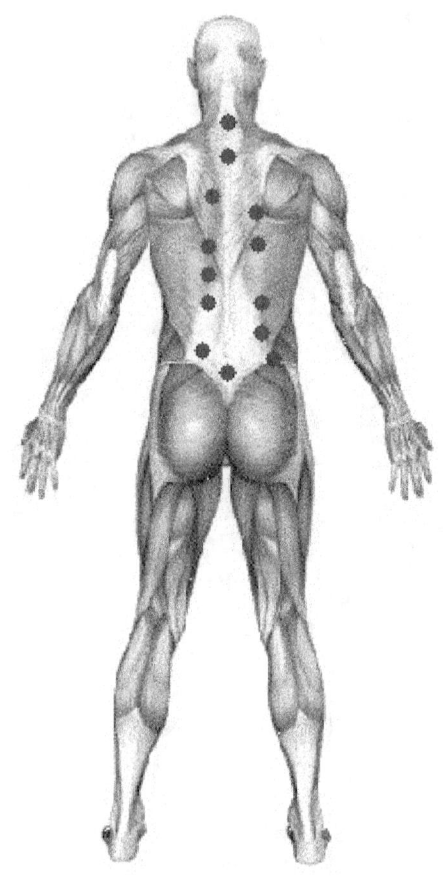

13 Cupping Points

63) Cupping for Full Paralysis

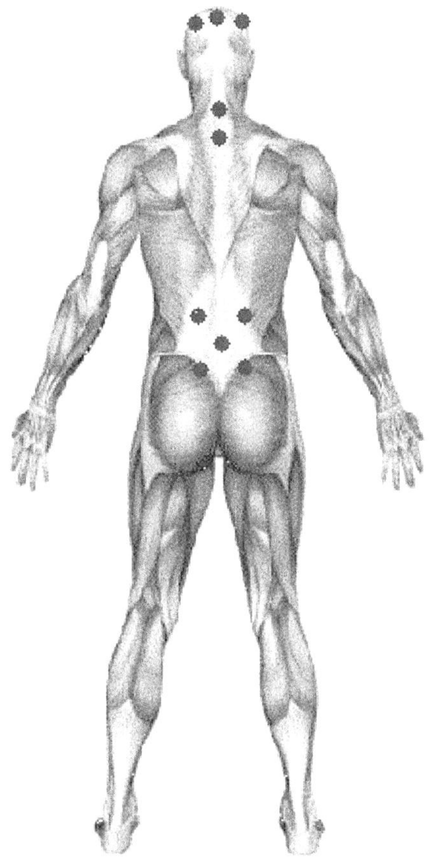

10 Cupping Points

64) Cupping for Stomach Disorder

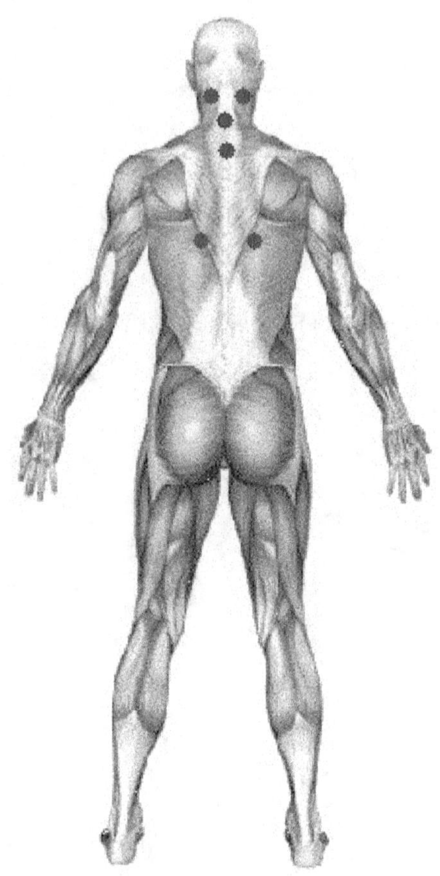

6 Cupping Points

65) Cupping for Chronic Coughing and Lung Diseases

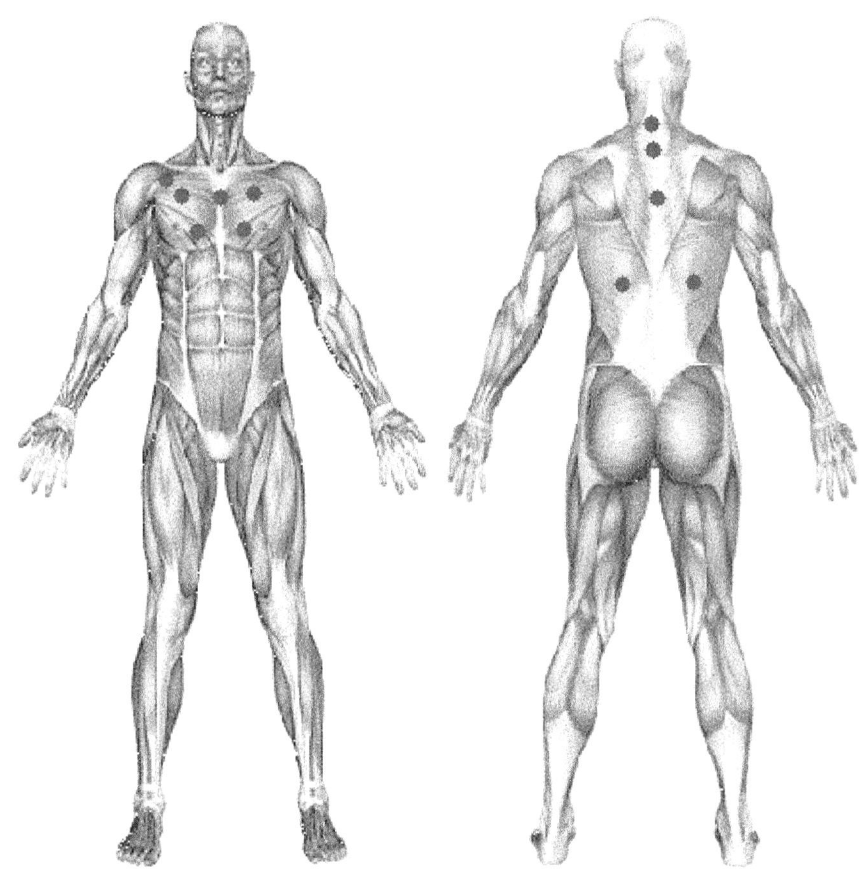

11 Cupping Points

66) Cupping for Prostate Disorder and Impotence

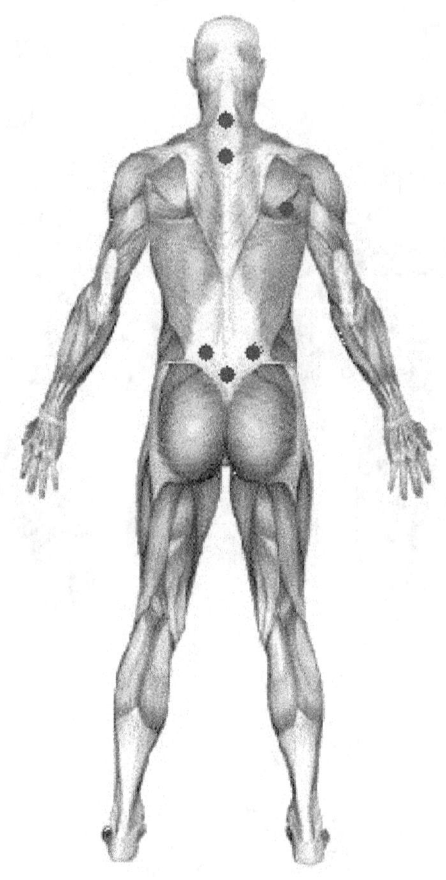

6 Cupping Points

67) Cupping for Coldness on the Soles of the Feet

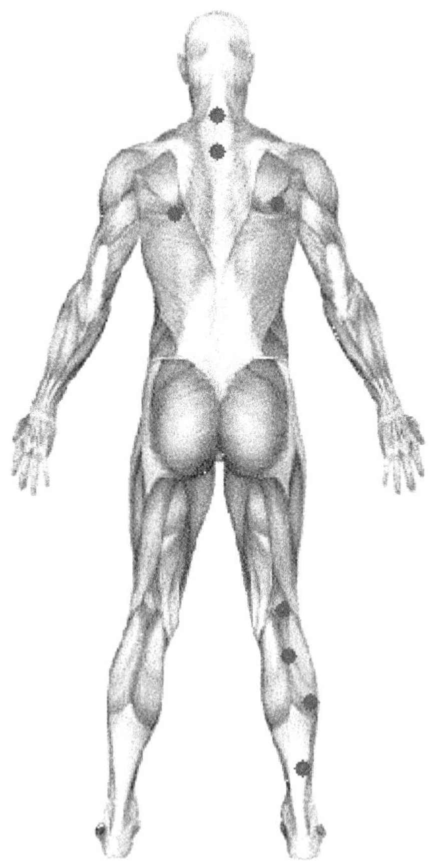

8 Cupping Points

68) Cupping for Pins and Needles in the Legs

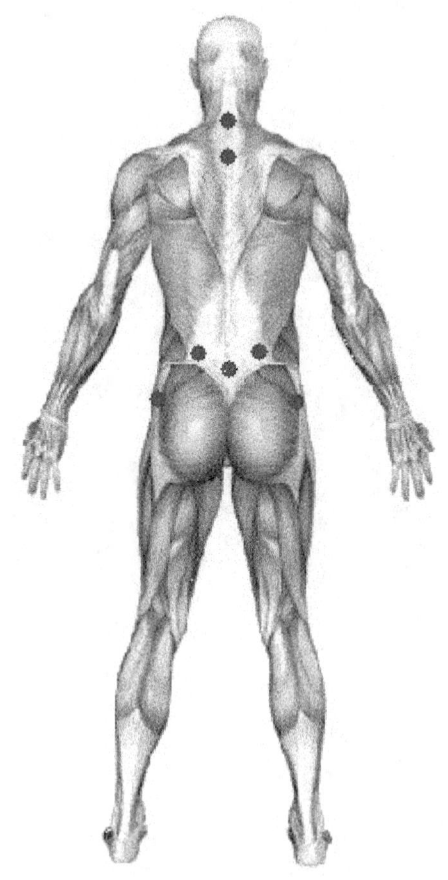

7 Cupping Points

69) Cupping for Pins and Needles in the Hands

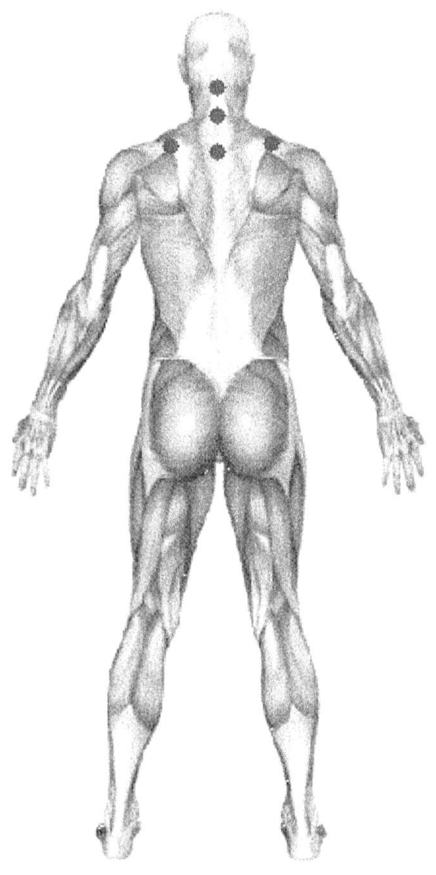

5 Cupping Points

70) Cupping for Muscle Pull (Sprain)

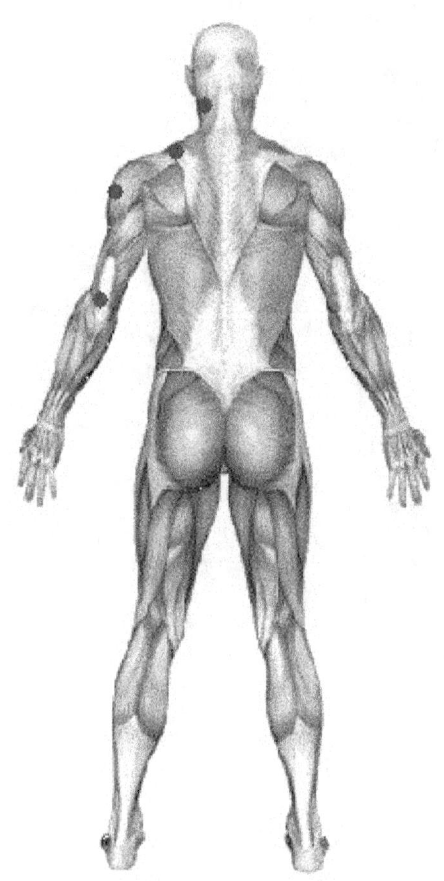

4 Cupping Points

71) Cupping for Brain Tumour

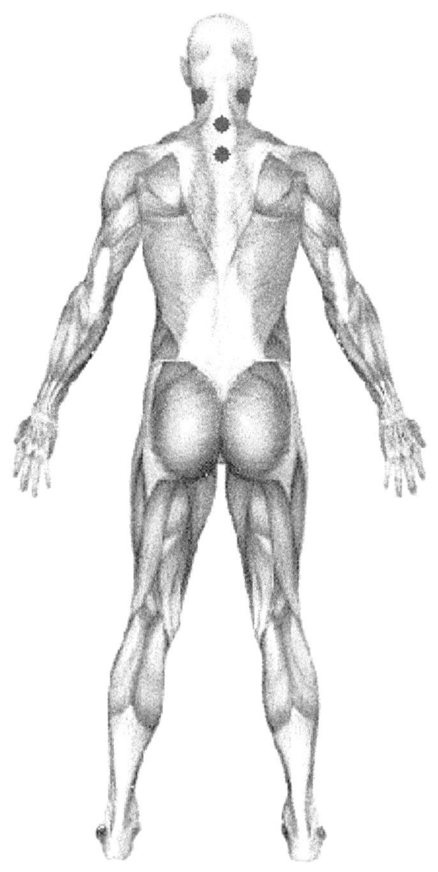

4 Cupping Points

72) Cupping for Thickening and Hardening of the Soles of the Feet

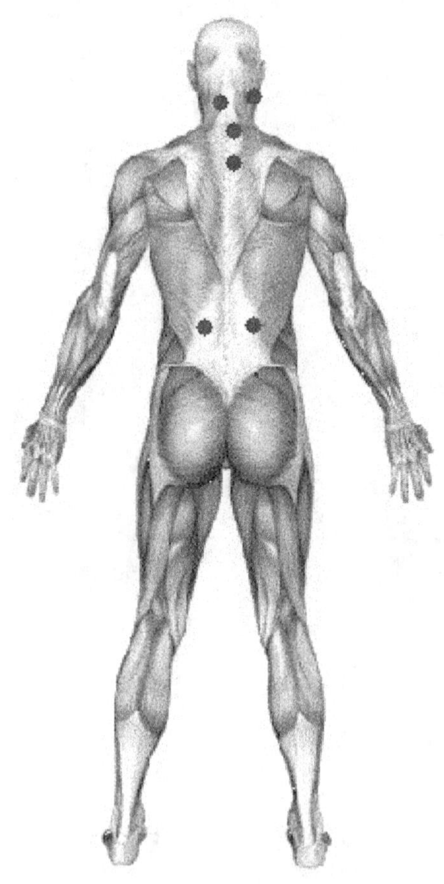

6 Cupping Points

73) Cupping for Numb Knees

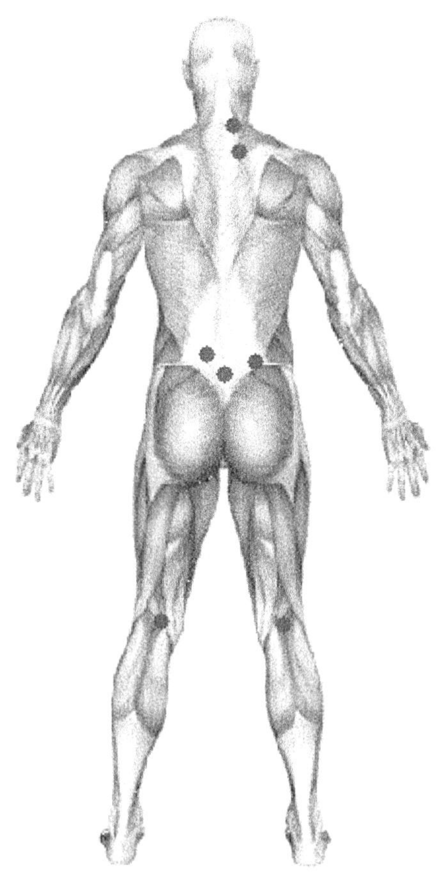

7 Cupping Points

74) Cupping for Pancreas Disorder

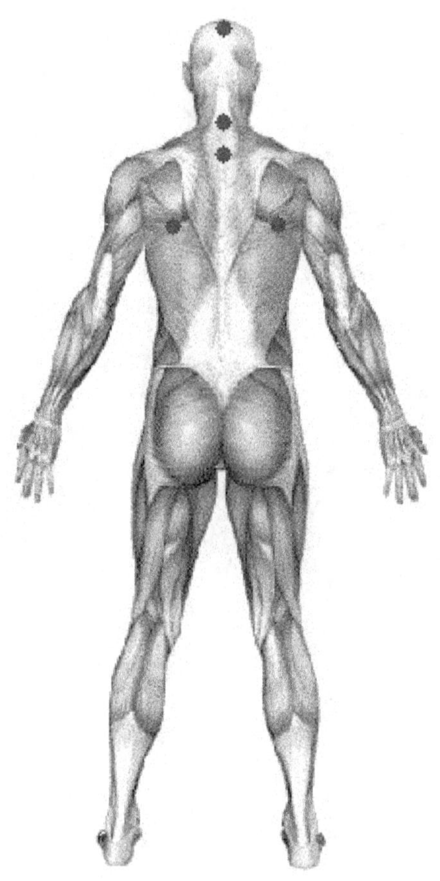

5 Cupping Points

75) Cupping for Backbone Disorder

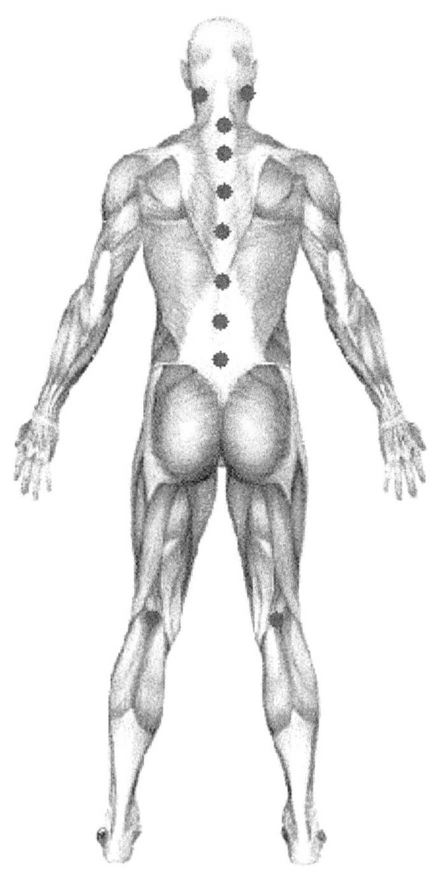

9 Cupping Points

76) Cupping for Bladder and Liver Disorders

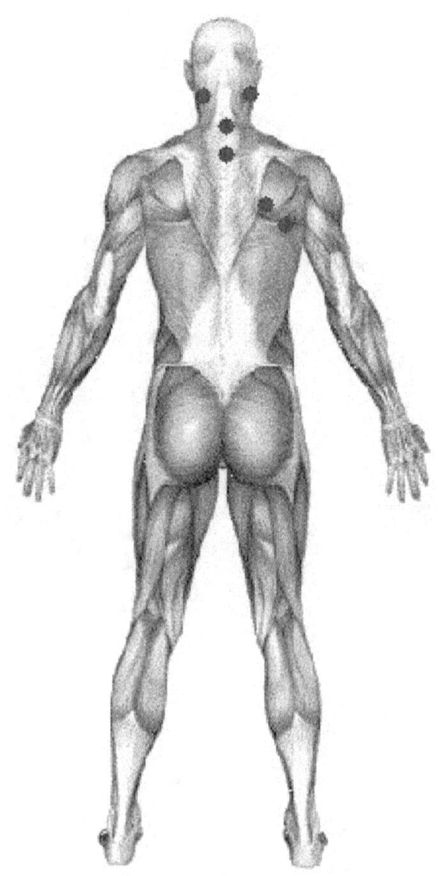

6 Cupping Points

77) Cupping for Period Pain for Women

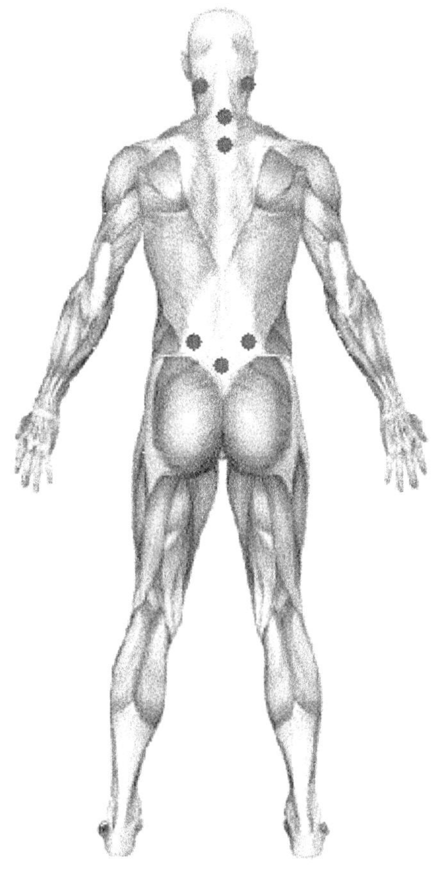

7 Cupping Points

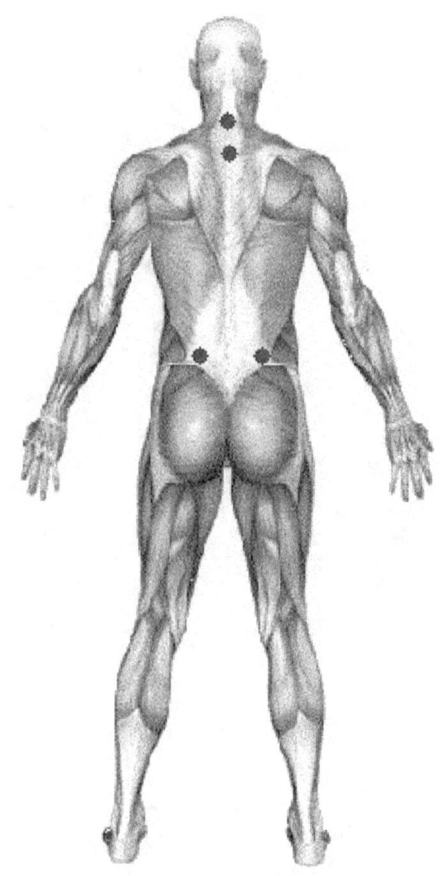

4 Cupping Points

79) Cupping for Nervousness, Tense and Restlessness

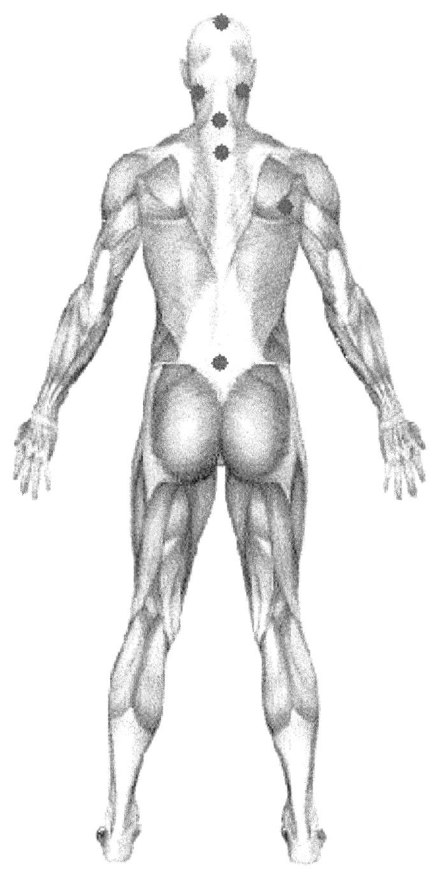

7 Cupping Points

80) Cupping for Weak Brain Cells Function

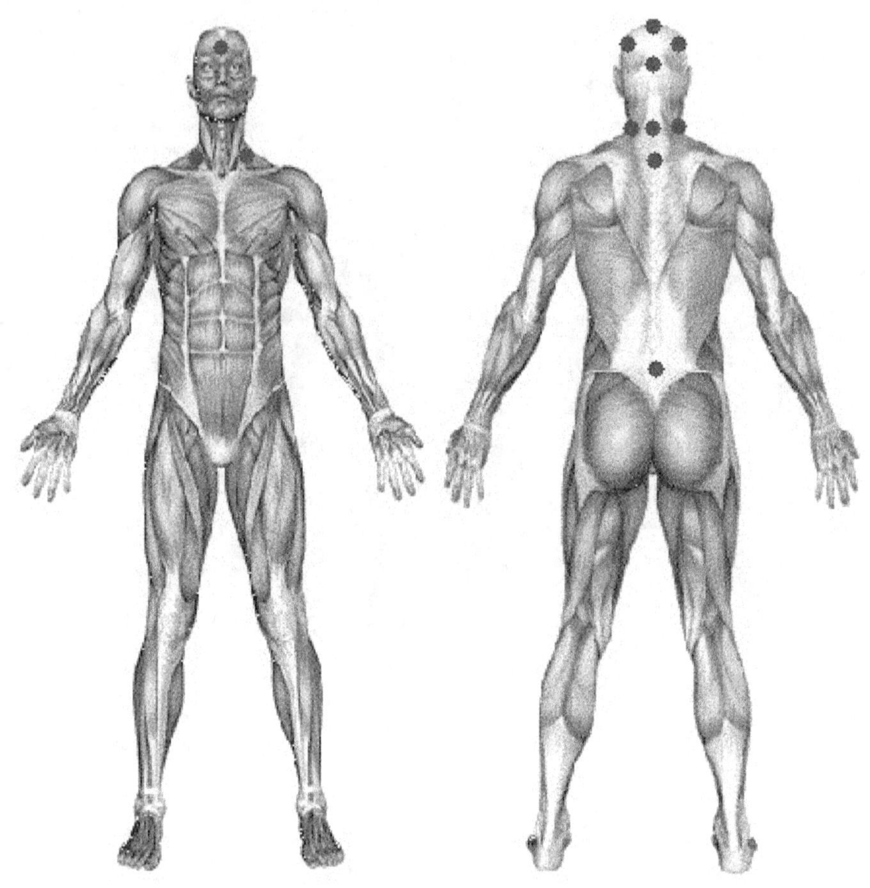

12 Cupping Points

81) Cupping for Ceased Menstruation

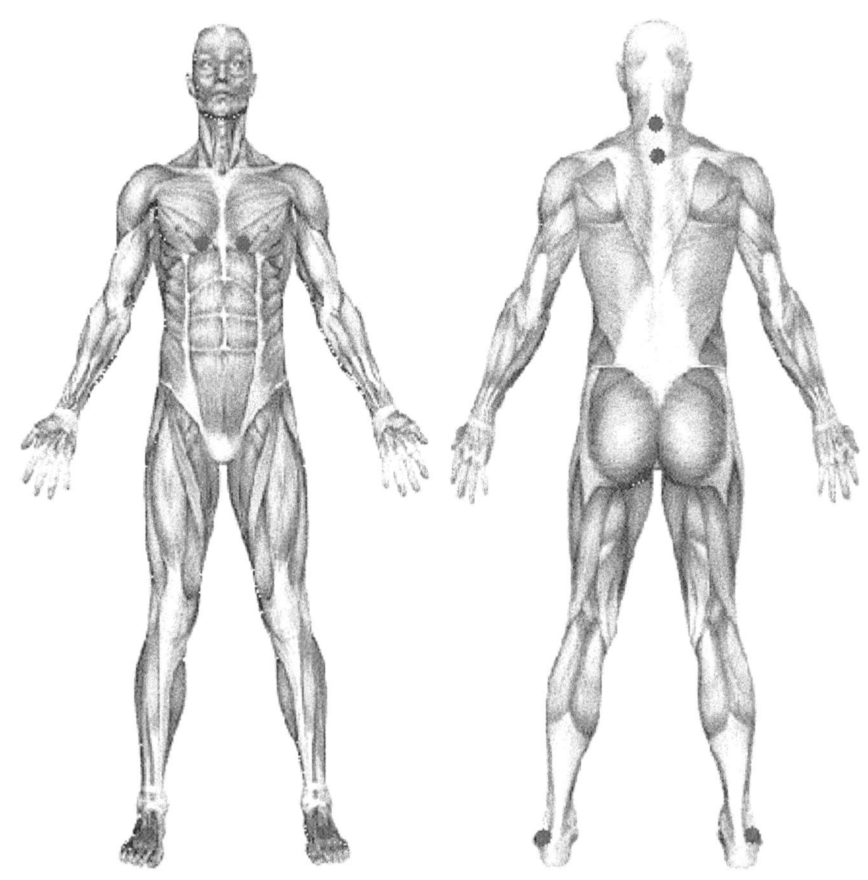

8 Cupping Points

82) Cupping for Testis Swelling

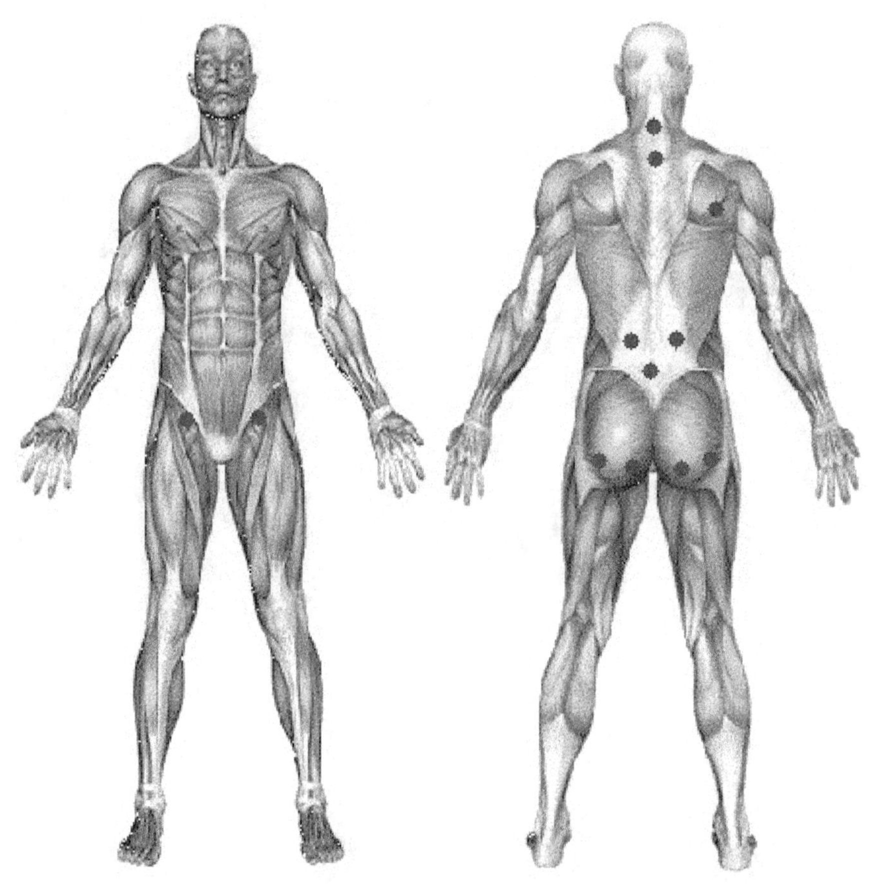

12 Cupping Points

83) Cupping for Cramps

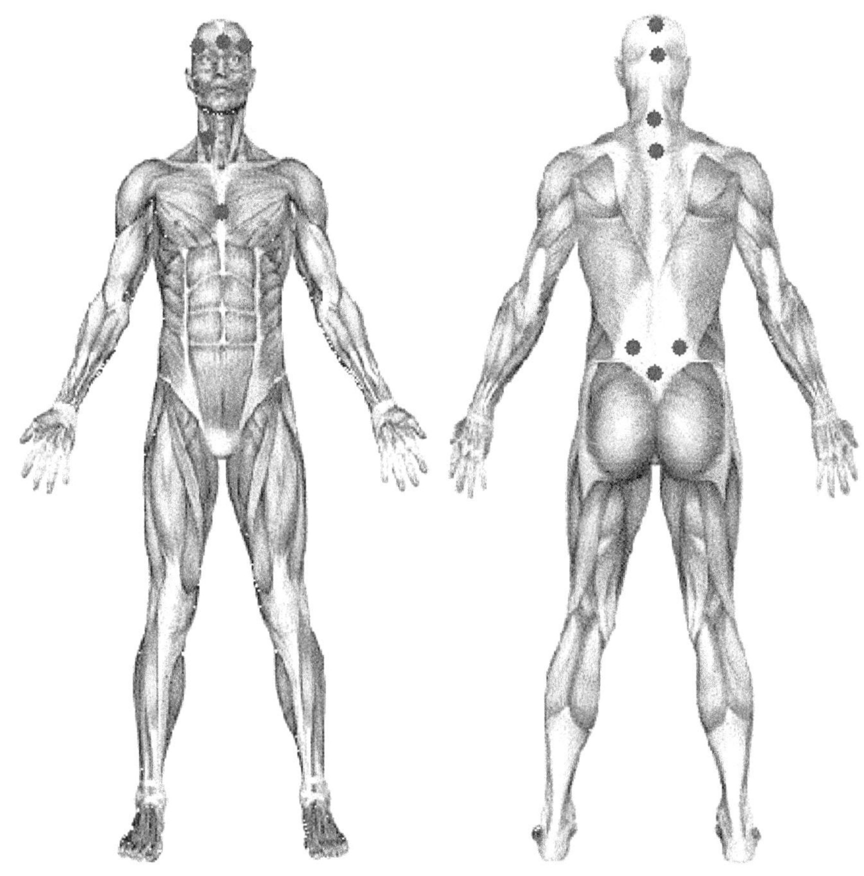

12 Cupping Points

84) Cupping for Unable to Speak

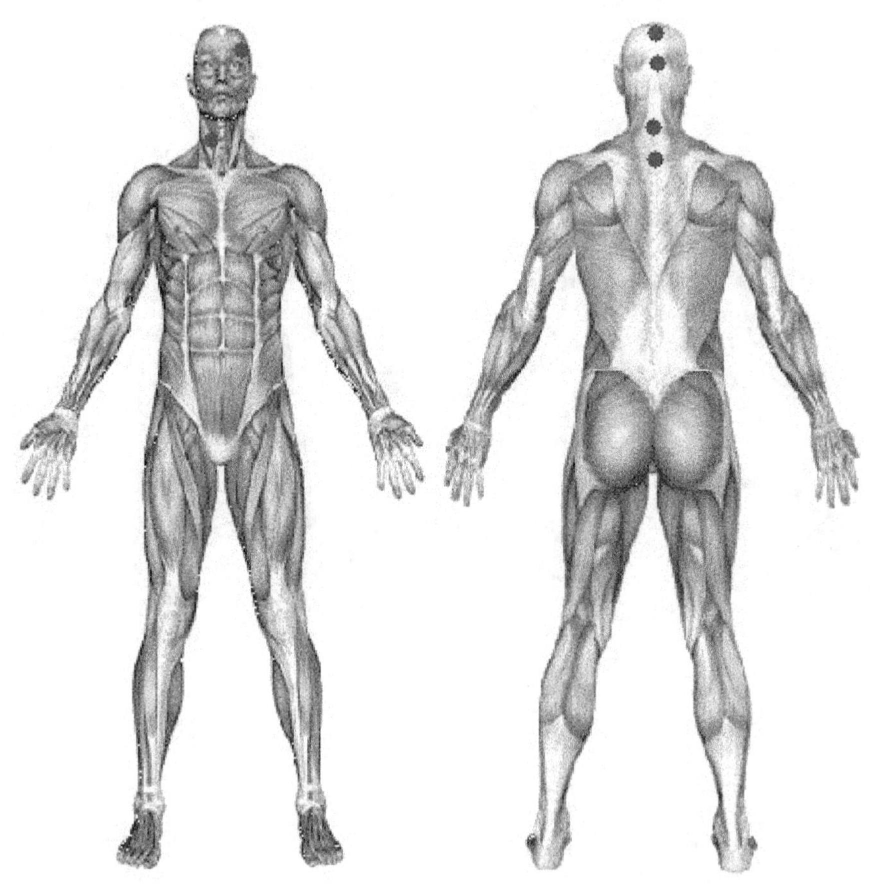

6 Cupping Points

85) Cupping for Eye Disease

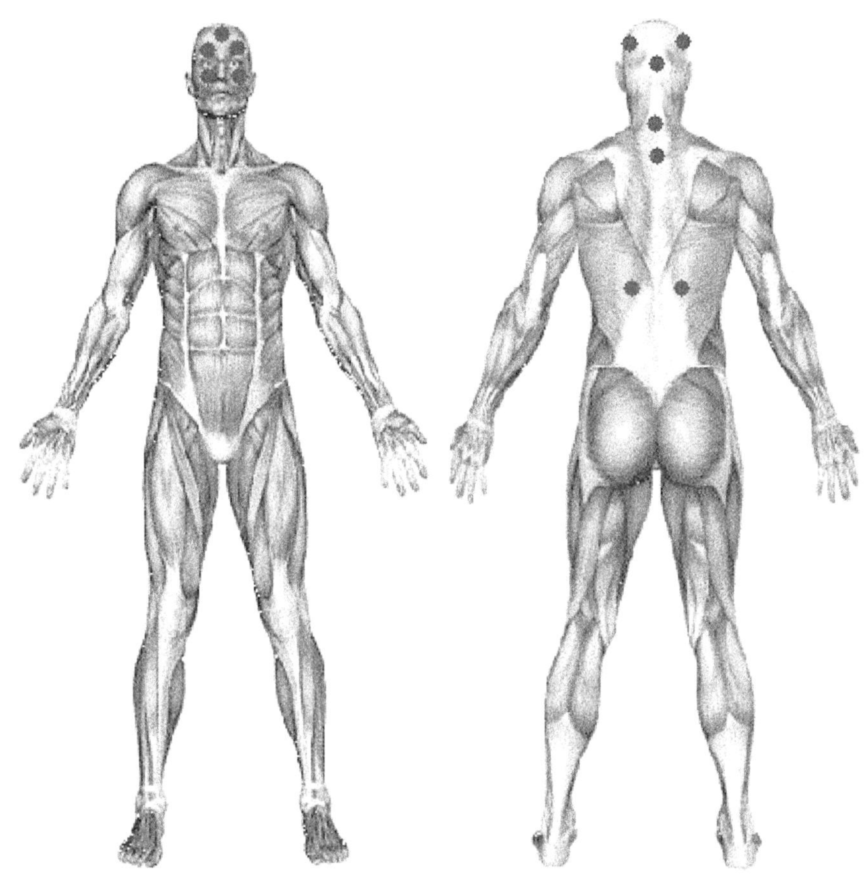

12 Cupping Points

86) Cupping for Vaginal Fluid Discharge

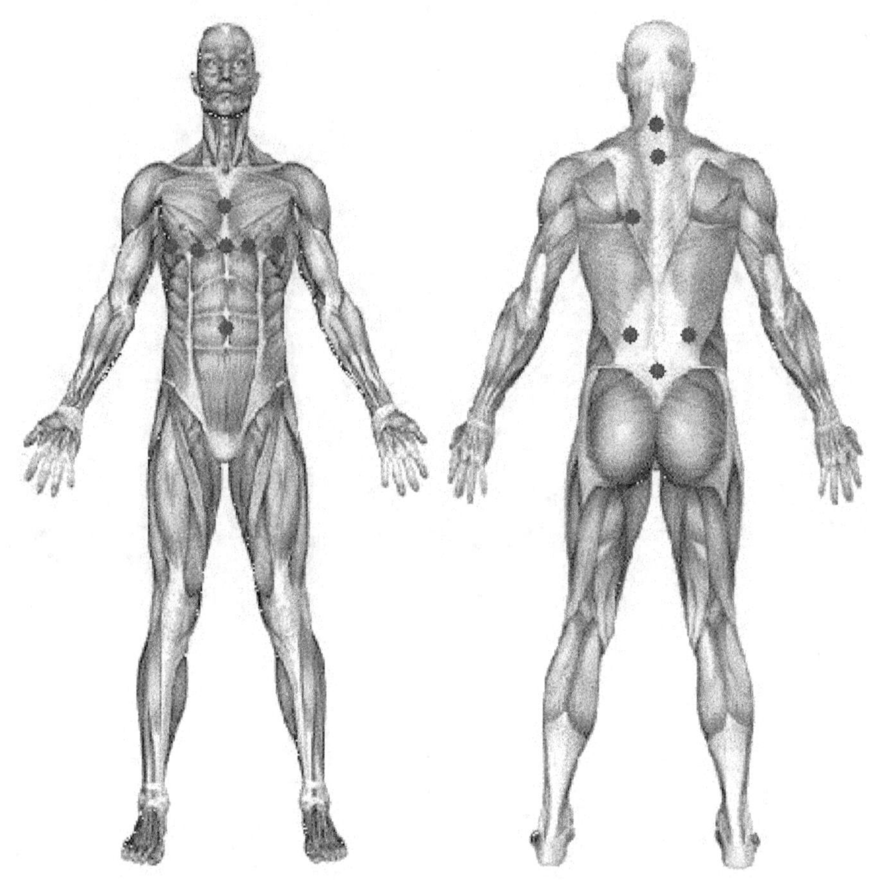

13 Cupping Points

87) Cupping for Nerve Inflammation

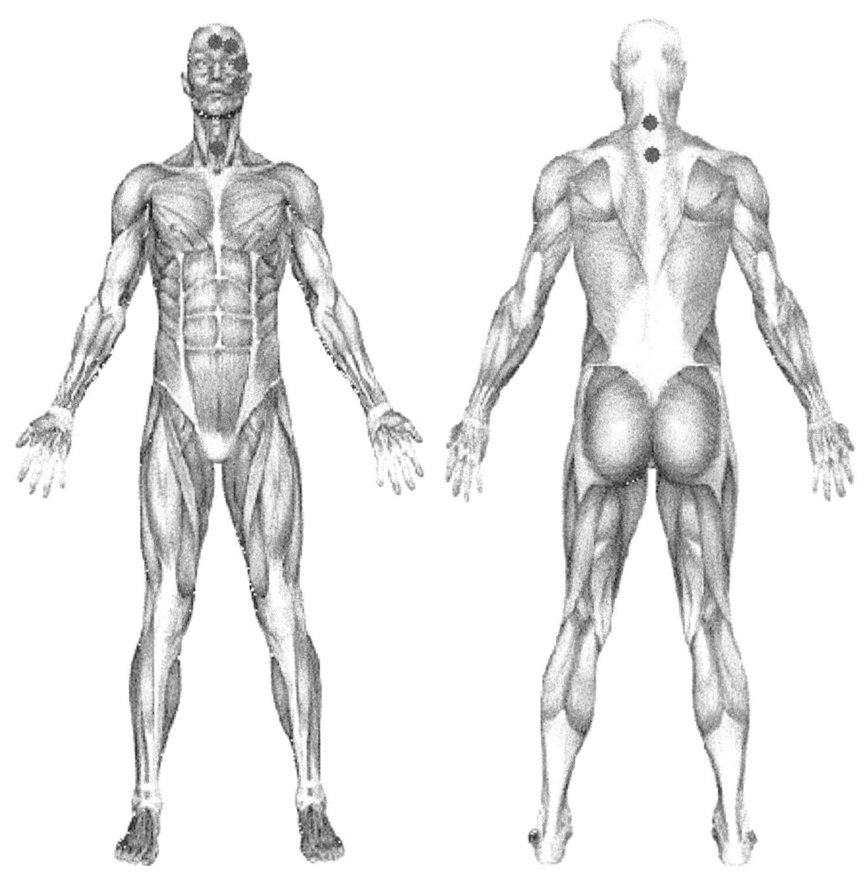

7 Cupping Points

88) Cupping for Fertility

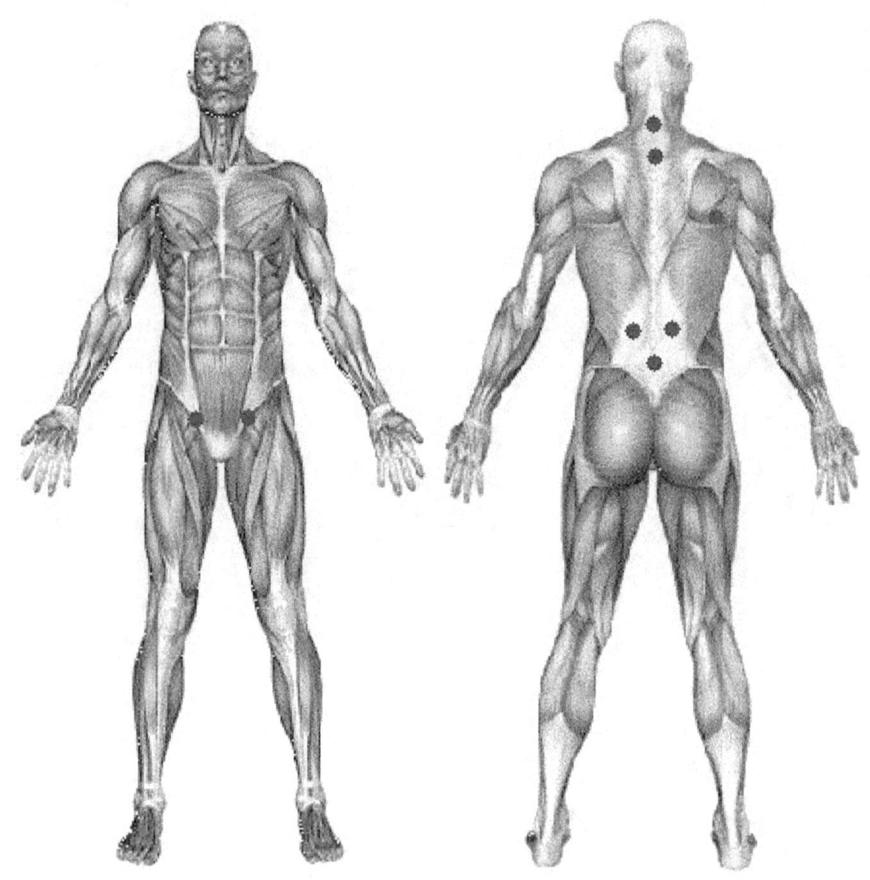

8 Cupping Points

89) Cupping for Low Blood Pressure

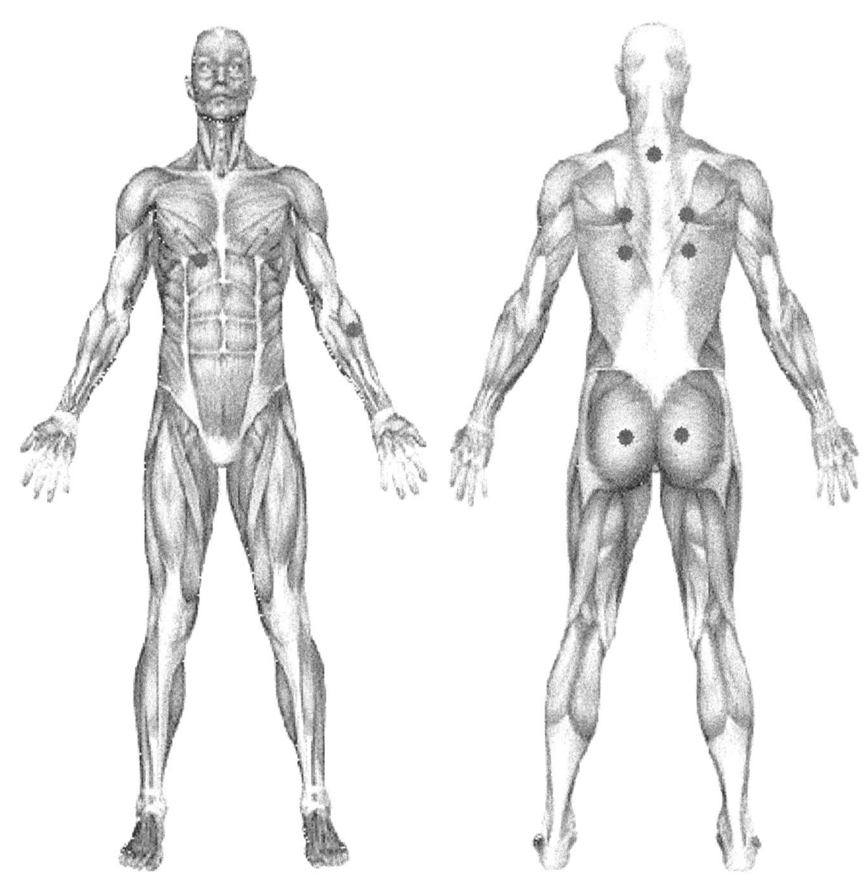

9 Cupping Points

90) Cupping for Womb-Related Diseases

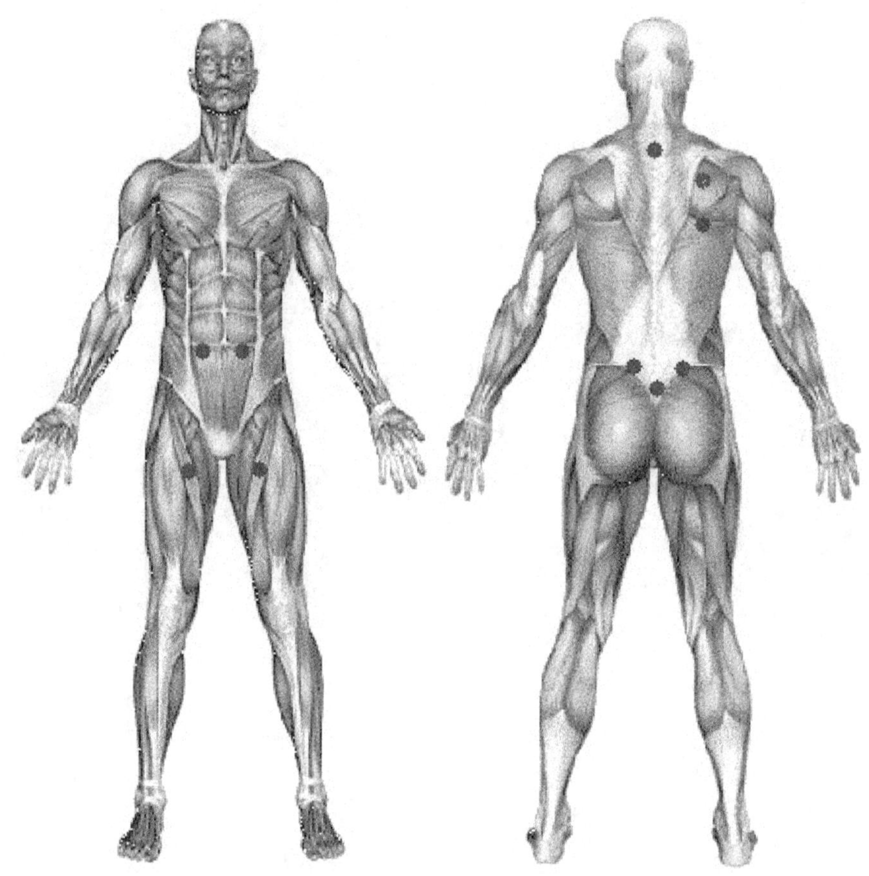

10 Cupping Points

91) Cupping for Eye Problems

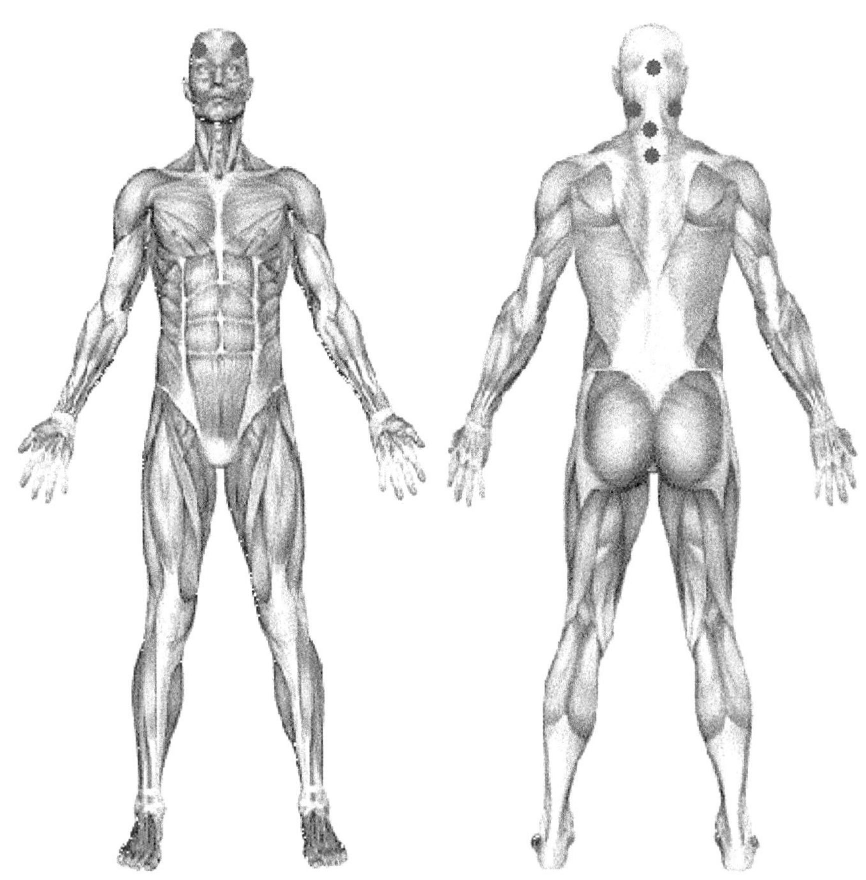

7 Cupping Points

92) Cupping for Headache due to Inflammation around the Nasal Cavity

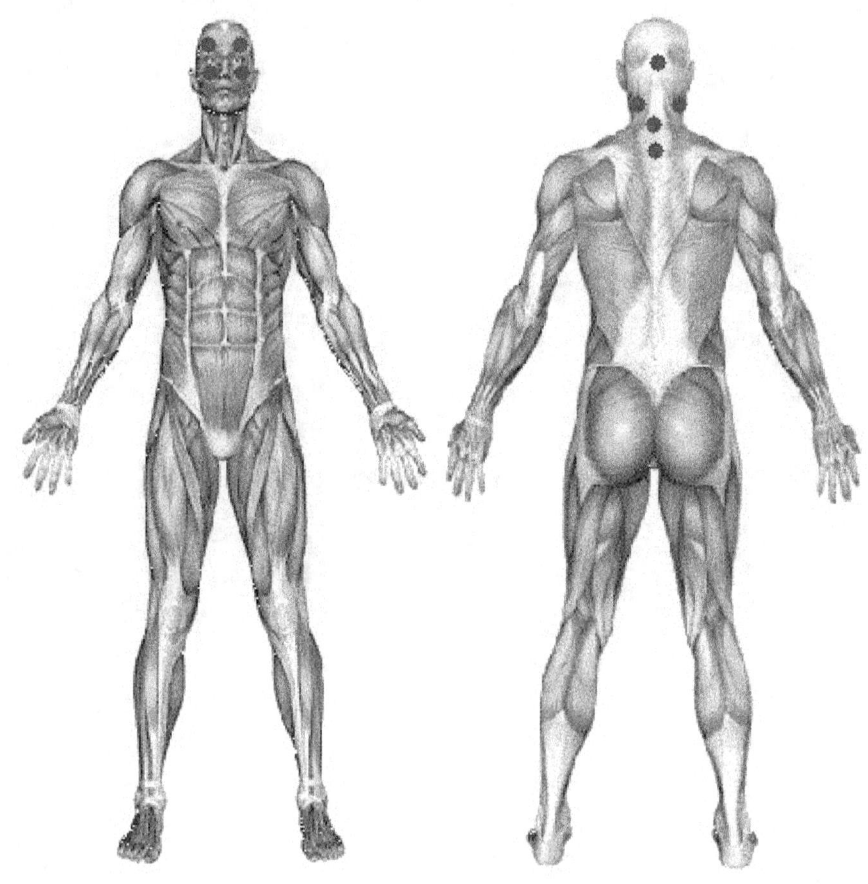

9 Cupping Points

93) Cupping for Anaemia

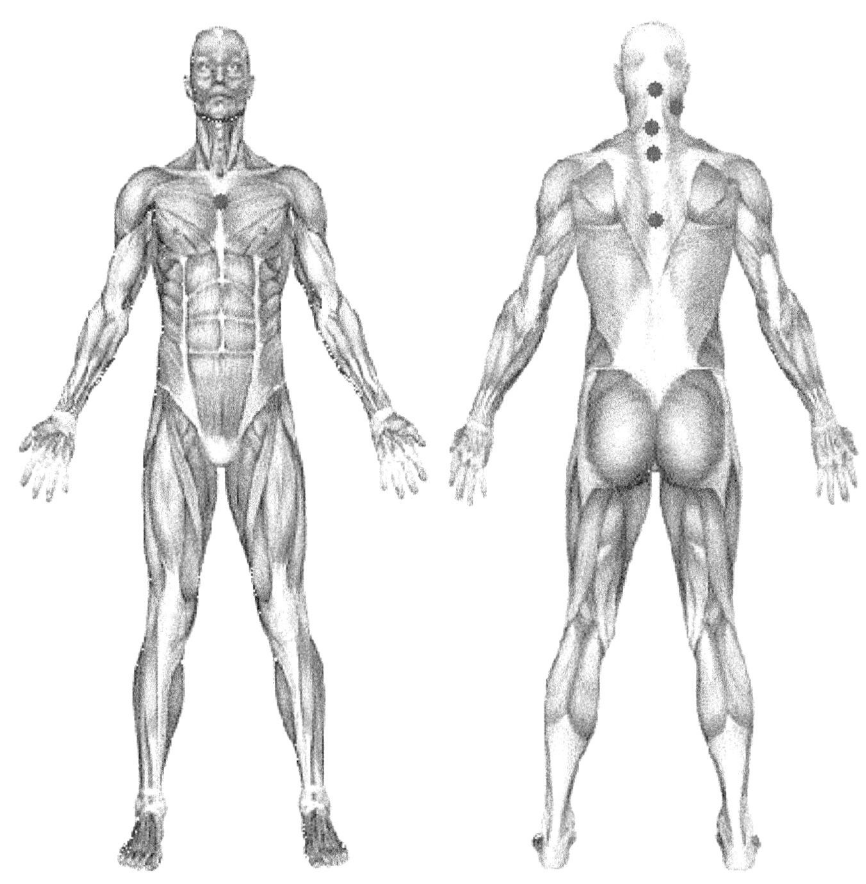

6 Cupping Points

94) Cupping for Influenza

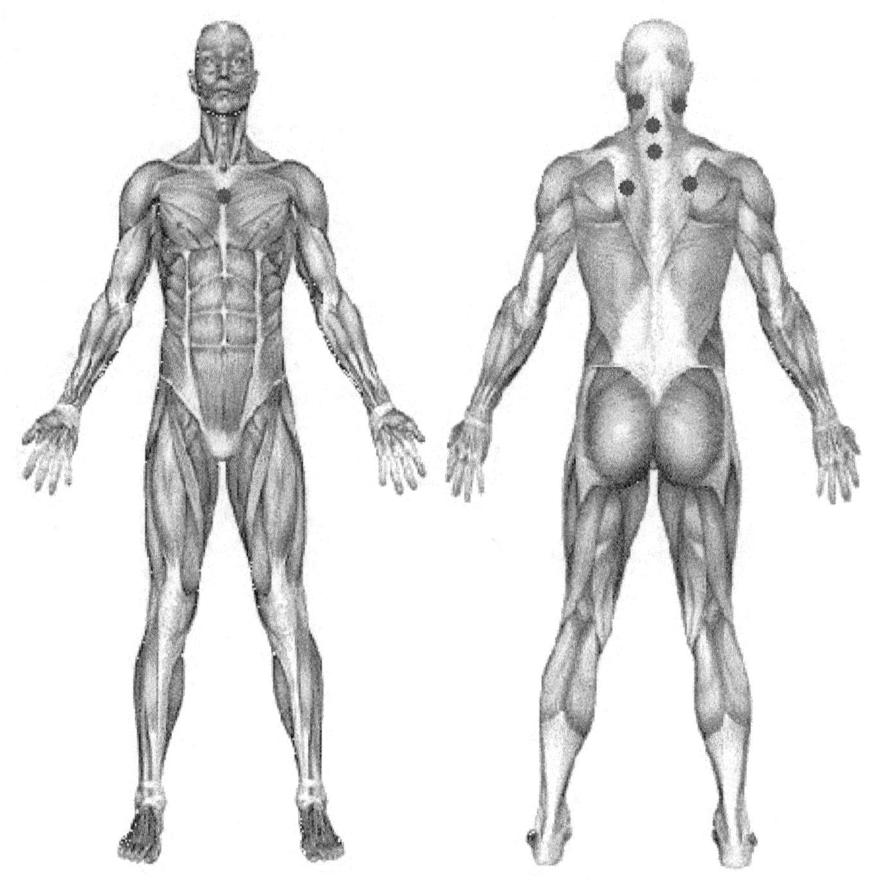

7 Cupping Points

THE END